Quick Review of
INI-CET

Institute of National Importance
Combined Entrance Test

MAY-2023 SUPPLEMENT

Authentic Questions with Explanations

Kamal KV
MBBS, MS (Orthopedics)

Foreign (Academic) Trips (Countries and Cities)

Georgia (Tbilisi, Batumi)
Russia (Nalchik, Cheboksary, Stavropol, Kazan)
Kyrgyzstan (Jalalabad, Osh, Bishkek)
Nepal (Bharatpur, Bhairahawa, Dharan)
Ukraine (Vinnytsia, Kiev)
China (Ningbo, Nanchang, Nanning, Dali, Fuzhou, Guangzhou)
Belarus (Minsk)
Kazakhstan (Almaty)

Peepee Publishers and Distributors (P) Ltd.®

Quick Review of INI-CET

May-2023 Supplement

Published by
Pawaninder P. Vij and Anupam Vij

Peepee Publishers and Distributors (P) Ltd.
Head Office: 160, Shakti Vihar, Pitam Pura, Delhi-110 034 (India)

Correspondence Address:

7/31, First Floor, Ansari Road, Daryaganj
New Delhi-110 002 (India)

Ph: 41512412, 23246245, 9811156083

e-mail: peepee160@yahoo.co.in

e-mail: peepee160@gmail.com

www.peepeepub.com

join us on facebook.com/pp.publishers

First Edition: 2023

ISBN: 978-81-9523-449-3

DEDICATION

This title is dedicated to all the (past and present) students of **drkamalkv's classes for FMGE**.

It is their faith and support, which is helping me in surviving this competitive world of coaching.

I started my classes in December 2011, and by God's grace and students support, I am still going on, singly.

I teach all the subjects singly (students call it **1-man Army**) and theoretically it seems very difficult to teach all subjects singly, but the unconditional support and faith of my dear students had made it practically possible.

drkamalkv

WhatsApp: 84 7000 4333
E-mail: drkamalkvgroup@gmail.com

SPECIAL THANKS

I would like to convey my heartfelt thanks to all those, who had arranged or served me during my foreign (academic) trips.

S. No.	*Countries*	*College*	*Timeline*
1.	**Georgia**	*i. Tbilisi*	Feb. 2018
		ii. Batumi	Feb. 2018
2.	**Russia**	*iii. Nalchik*	Oct. 2018, Feb. 2019, Dec. 2019
		iv. Cheboksary	Oct. 2018, Dec. 2019
		v. Stavropol	March 2019
		vi. Kazan	March 2019
3.	**Kyrgyzstan**	*vii. Jalalabad*	Dec. 2018, May 2019, Dec. 2021, Dec. 2022
		viii. Osh	May 2019, Dec. 2022
		ix. Bishkek	Dec. 2022, April 2023
4.	**Nepal**	*x. Bhairahawa*	May 2019
		xi. Bharatpur	May 2019, Sep. 2019
		xii. Dharan	Sep. 2019
5.	**Ukraine**	*xiii. Vinnytsia*	Nov. 2019
		xiv. Kiev	Nov. 2019
6.	**China**	*xv. Ningbo*	Oct. 2018
		xvi. Nanchang	Nov. 2018
		xvii. Nanning	Nov. 2018
		xviii. Dali	Nov. 2018
		xix. Fuzhou	June 2019
		xx. Guangzhou	June 2019
7.	**Belarus**	*xxi. Minsk*	Jan. 2020
8.	**Kazakhstan**	*xxii. Almaty*	April 2023

drkamalkv

WhatsApp: 84 7000 4333

Facebook: drkamalkvgroup

PREFACE

I have written books for many medical exams (FMGE, UPSC–CMS, DNB and NEET–PG), but a book on AIIMS–PG (now INI–CET) was missing from my shelf. I feel very blessed to have this one also (finally ☺).

Usually, I can write a supplement kind of book within 1 month. However, for this particular title, it took nearly three months. In initial few weeks, I could finalize only the format. I tried many formats, but the current one was more satisfying and a somewhat new pattern.

The presentation of this title is very unique, and of course student-friendly. As we, all know that for AIIMS–PG/INI–CET exams, one should have thorough knowledge of the topic. Keeping this fact in mind, I have tried to compile relevant explanation for the question.

Salient features of this title:

1. **Key points:** Wherever I felt that discussion of the options is not providing enough details about the topic as such, I have created this another heading to summarize important points about the main topic.
2. **Let's discuss the options:** I have tried to explain all the four options. Why one of the option is the answer and why others are not. The options are discussed in relation to the question.
3. **Coming back to the question:** Instead of writing the answer directly, I have employed an indirect approach to mention the answer (as a statement).

As I always say, students are the best judge of an author's work. In addition, I personally feel, there is always enough room left for further improvement. Therefore, I expect my dear students to share their valuable feedbacks regarding the betterment of subsequent editions.

Despite my best efforts, some errors must have crept in. Since I have typed the entire content myself, I expect a few spelling mistakes. I request dear readers, to share the same with me (on the channels mentioned below).

Until now, students had supported all my titles. I hope the same kind of response for this title too.

Errata of this title (if any) would be updated on my **telegram** channel **(drkamalkvgroup)**.

Please do join this channel for other relevant updates as well.

Hope this title will serve its purpose.

15 August 2023

drkamalkv

WhatsApp: 84 7000 4333
Android App: drkamalkvgroup

ACKNOWLEDGEMENTS

Every one of us is blessed in some or other way and I feel, I am born to write books☺. I am an orthopedic surgeon but honestly, I do not enjoy much my clinical practice or even making You-tube videos. I love to read textbooks and learn as much as possible. Probably this tendency had helped me in teaching all subjects singly to Foreign Medical Graduates. Even for this title, I have studied a lot of matter. One more thing, I do all the type work and designing by myself. I try to be creative in writing books. I try to present the content in a unique and of course, in a student-friendly manner. Readers will appreciate this fact, when they will go through this book. Therefore, I must thank Almighty for blessing me this unique talent.

I started my journey as an author in 2011, when I wrote the book for Foreign Medical Graduate Examination/FMGE. Since then, I never looked back and whenever any publisher approached for me a title, I grabbed the opportunity with both the hands. This is my passion for writing books, that I was able to cross the 50th title mark long back. Therefore, thanks are due for my publishers, who had given me the platform to highlight my talent.

In this title, I have tried to explain all the four options. There were two instances, which made me follow this approach.

i. Firstly, one of the reader left a review for my NEET–PG 2022 supplement that explanations are concise, and he feel unsatisfied with those concise explanations. He pointed out that why only the option (related to answer) is discussed and why not the other options.

ii. Secondly, when I was working in Allen NExT, my boss (and one of my best friends), *Dr. Sarvejeet Singh sir* (Academic Director, Allen NExT) told me to solve the question bank explaining all the four options. Unfortunately, I could not continue longer in Allen NExT, but that idea remained in my mind.

For past three months, I was so much involved in this book that I literally did nothing else. I did not worked anywhere. This made me face financial crisis at times. I am highly thankful to few persons who lend me money during my tough times. This include my father *Hony. Capt/AEC ML Verma*, my brother *Engr.*

Anil Verma, my sister *Deeptii Karan*, my best friend *Dr. Ahmed Dawar*, my ex-students *Dr. Soumik Mukherjee* and *Dr. Firoj Khan*. I am highly thankful to my tenants, *Dr. Ajay, Dr. Ravi* and *Dr. Sehdev* too, for paying the rent timely☺. This helped me in sustaining through my tough time.

I feel highly thankful to my friends *Dr. Vinod Singh* (DMS, ESI Hospital) and *Dr. Lalit Verma* (ENT specialist) as well.

Apart from this, there are many people, whom I do not know personally, but they have always wished for my well-being. This includes my ex-students, their family members, my ex-patients etc. I pay a big thanks to all of them.

Usually I like to do all my work singly. Therefore, I do not have acknowledgment in that terms, that who helped me in writing books. I can just mention the names of the person, who helped me indirectly (as a human).

I convey my thanks to:

- Almighty (for imparting me with this passion of writing books and teaching).
- My parents (for imparting qualities of a good human being)
- My brothers and sister (for giving me some wonderful memories of childhood).
- My wife (for supporting me in all my endeavors).
- My daughters (for allowing me to use their share of time for my academic work); and
- My dear students (for accepting all my titles with equal enthusiasm and also, who made me academically strong).

Special thanks to **Mr. Pawaninder Paul Vij** and **Mr. Anupam Vij** for accepting all my work, without any hesitancy or objection.

Thanks are due for everyone behind this project from the publication house, especially Mr. S.K. Sharma and Mr. Pawan Sharma.

drkamalkv

WhatsApp: 84 7000 4333
Website: www.drkamalkvgroup.co.in

AN IDEAL WAY TO SCORE GOOD IN INI-CET EXAMINATION

In the following paragraphs, I will sum up some important factors which should be considered for optimum result.

First crucial factor is 'Time': One has only 6 months (theoretically) to prepare and 20 subjects to cover (considering every subject as a separate one).

Now, even in this period, the initial one month is not used for studies by most of the students.

Freshers may use the initial time for searching the best coaching classes/online app/study matter and so on.

Similarly, after the result, the people who could not make it need some time to overcome the setbacks and prepare themselves again for the exam.

Therefore, talking in practical terms, only 4–5 months are available for studies.

Second important factor is 'What to study'?: There are no definitive guidelines regarding the content and the depth of studies.

Since this is an AIIMS level examination, you have to literally read everything and that too in detail.

Instead of chasing after many books/app, please choose one (with which you are comfortable) and go through it keeping the time restrictions in mind. The better example is that there are plenty of students, who just read one particular app since beginning, and came up with excellence.

Going through the past years, MCQs bank is of utmost importance for every exam, and for this one too. Needless to say, previous years MCQ bank gives you an idea that which all topics (at least) you need to be perfect with.

Third important factor is 'How to study'?: Make sure you cover the syllabus in detail at least once and two revisions (up to this much is practically possible). Anything studied is of no use unless and until it is revised.

When you are going through the things in detail, just mark the important things/confusing things, and revise only these things during the revision phase. Similarly, while reading MCQs, put a cross in front of those MCQs which you can answer very easily (it means you do not need to revise them again).

Revising the matter, which you know very well, is often suicidal. It gives you a false feeling as if you know too much and, secondly and more importantly, consumes a lot of time.

It is not practically possible to revise everything. Therefore, some segregation needs to be done. Starting from day 1 of your preparation, that what all content you have to revise later.

So, give the initial three months for detailed study and revise the important (segregated) things in the subsequent two months.

One important factor, please 'be positive' in your approach while preparing. For clearing an examination, you need to have two important things: Self-belief, that yes, I have the potential and I will definitely score well in the exam.

I can sense the amount of psychological pressure on the students, and with such a big burden on your chest, it is very difficult to get rid of this feeling, but still try to overcome this fear.

It will definitely help you in performing well in the examination hall.

Most important factor is 'What is your approach in the examination hall'? You may have prepared well but until and unless you apply your knowledge in examination hall, everything is a sheer waste.

So, enter the examination hall with a positive note. Say to yourself repeatedly, 'I have prepared well and I am going to perform well'.

Lastly, the crucial factor is 'How do you solve the paper'? I advise the students to divide the time slot into three parts. Now let us discuss, what is this **3 phases theory** of solving the paper in the examination hall.

Total duration of the examination (3 hours/180 minutes) can be divided into 3 parts of 75 minutes, 75 minutes and 30 minutes respectively. You can change the values as per your calculation.

In the **first 75 minutes**, read all the questions properly. Try to mark out the negative statements, like Except, False, etc. In addition, read the MCQ statements properly and get to know what actually is asked. Do not be in any haste, as it may lead to errors. Say, for example, the questions may be like this: 'In Wilson's disease, what is being used for management'. A student in haste/panic may not understand the things properly, may presume that the question asks about the substance deposited in Wilson's disease, and will mark the answer as Copper (whereas the right answer is Zinc). In this phase, one should be able to solve the simplest questions (may be around 40–60), which need not much effort. Therefore, in first phase, read all the 200 MCQs and answer the simpler ones (one-liner kind of questions). Avoid solving calculation based, all-except or other questions which demand time and concentration.

The **next 75 minutes** are very crucial as in this time slot; you have to read the remaining (140–160) questions again with concentration. For many questions, you may have to think hard to get up to the proper answer. In this phase, you may come across many questions in which you may be confused between two options. Apply your knowledge to get to the most appropriate answer. This phase should be utilized for solving match the following, multiple correct options, all except kind of questions.

In the **last 30 minutes**, simply have a look at the answers you have marked, avoiding the tendency of changing the answers. It is a common observation that most of the times; we replace a right answer with wrong one.

In exams with negative marking, for some questions 'neglect' is a better choice than 'act'. If you don't know anything about the question, it's better you leave that question (unless you are aiming for top 10 rank). Guesswork should be applied to only those questions, where you can rule out two of the options.

This is my advice. You can modify the plan as per your convenience.

drkamalkv

WhatsApp: 84 7000 4333

WhatsApp Community: drkamalkvgroup

MY AMBITION

My grandparents always hoped that I should respect them as a 'good' grandson.

My parents wanted me to serve them as a 'good' son.

My brothers and sister wished that I should behave like a 'good' brother.

My wife dreamt that I should deal with her as a 'good' husband.

My daughters thought that I should take care of her like a 'good' father.

My teachers prayed that I should succeed like a 'good' student.

My students expected that I should teach them like a 'good' teacher.

However, I am striving hard to become a 'good' human being. Because, I know, the day I shall become a good human being, I shall imbibe all the abovementioned qualities within me.

drkamalkv

WhatsApp: 84 7000 4333

Skype id: drkamalkvgroup

CONTENTS

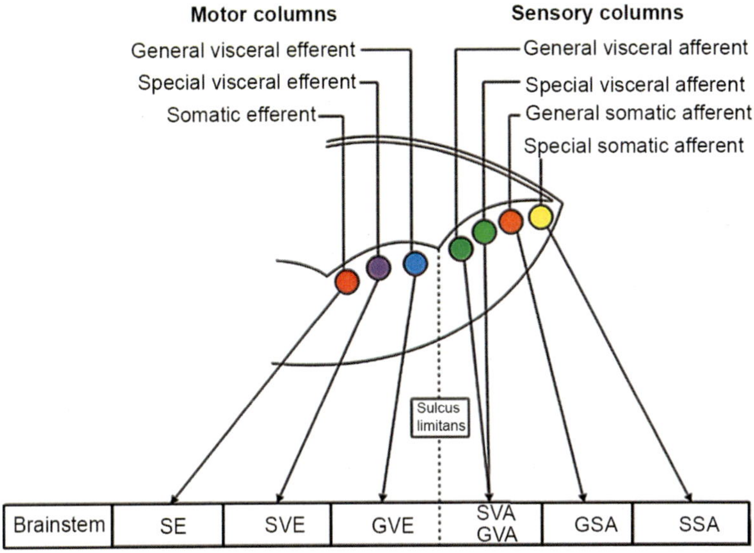

Page No. 5

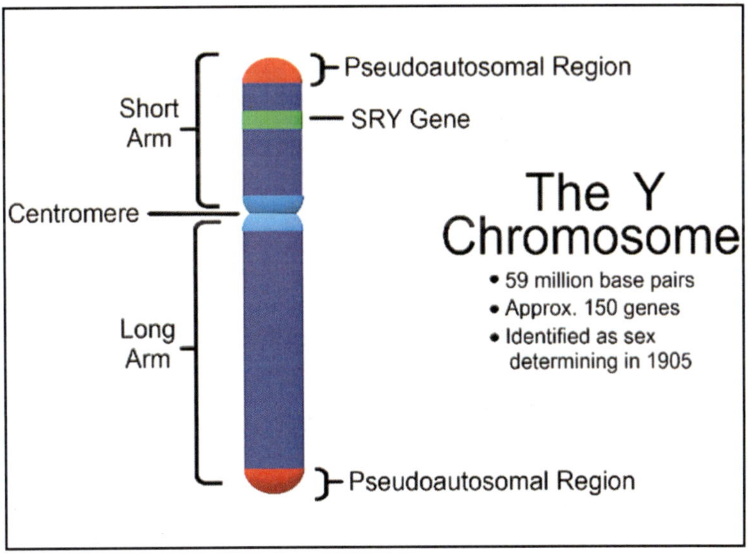

Page No. 11

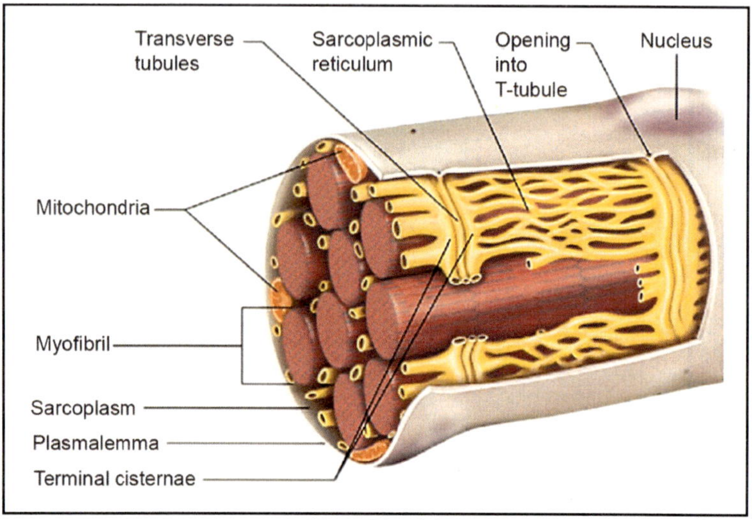

Page No. 14

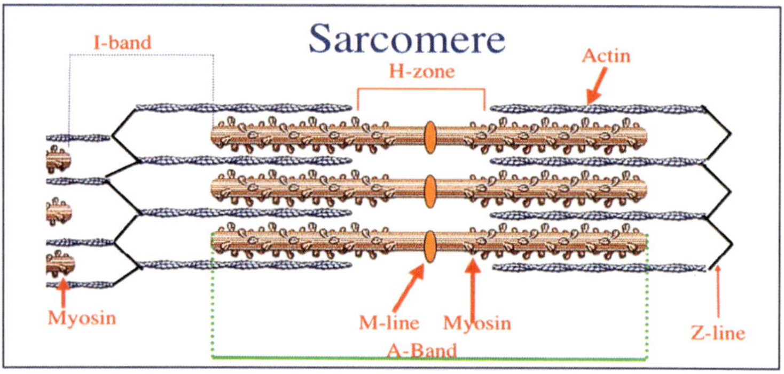

Page No. 24

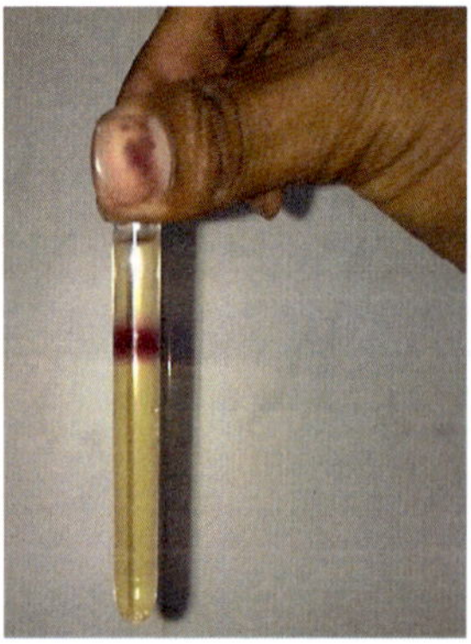

Page No. 29

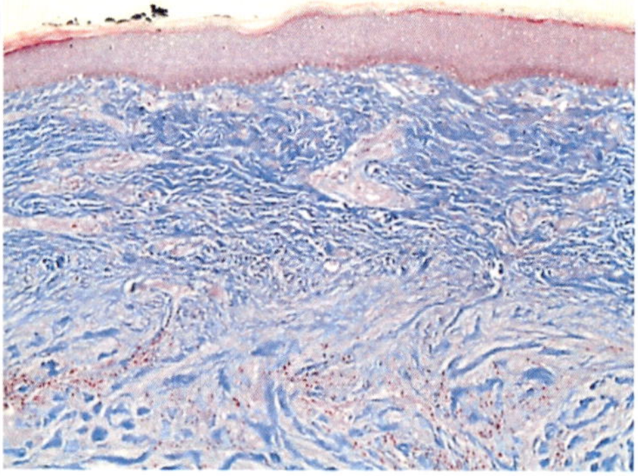

Page No. 49

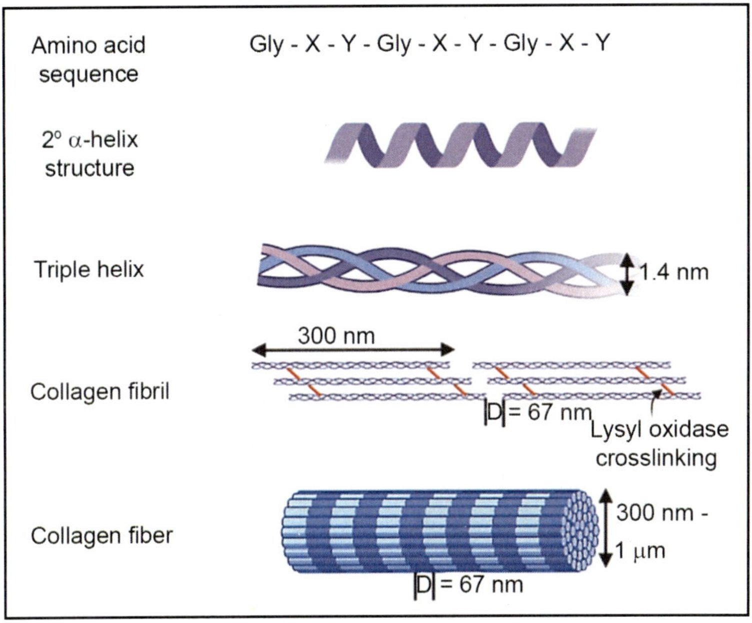

Page No. 38

Closure Color	Collection Tube	Mix by Inverting
	Blood Cultures	8 to 10 times
	Serum (glass tube)	—
	Citrate	3 to 4 times
	BD SST™ Gel Separator Tube	5 times
	BD SST Gel Separator Tube	"
	Serum (plastic tube)	"
	Heparin	8 to 10 times
	BD PST™ Gel Separator Tube With Heparin	"
	EDTA	8 to 10 times
	Fluoride (glucose tube)	8 to 10 times

Page No. 62

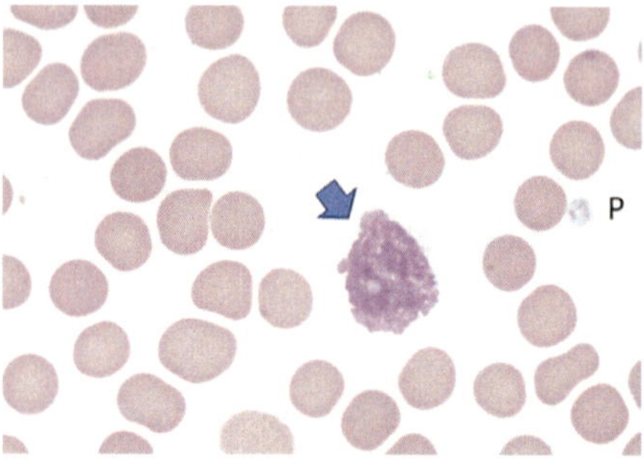

Page No. 51

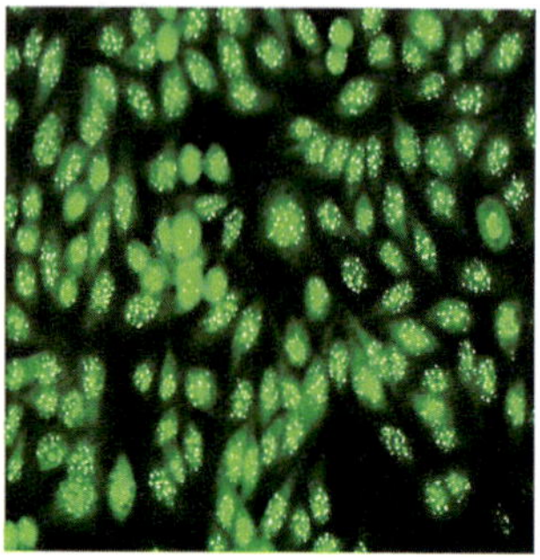

Page No. 67

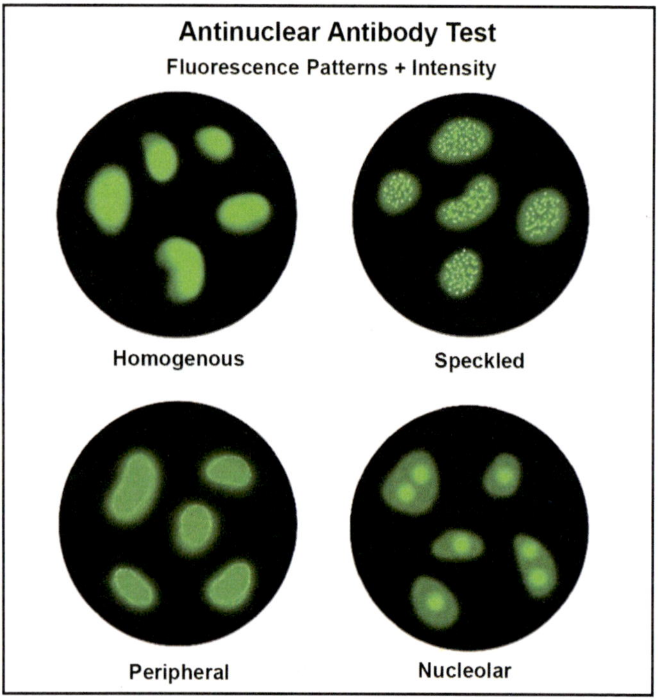

Page No. 68

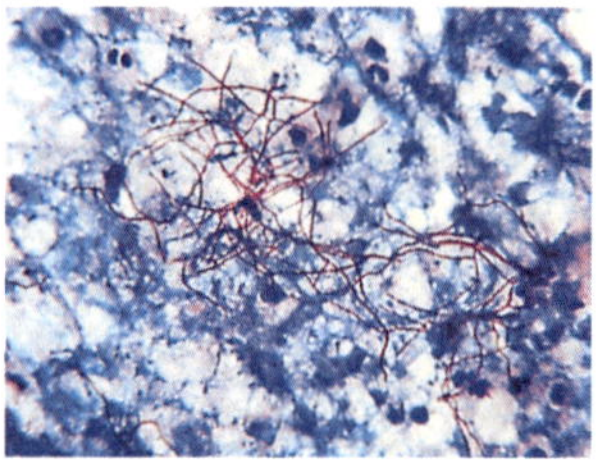

Page No. 84

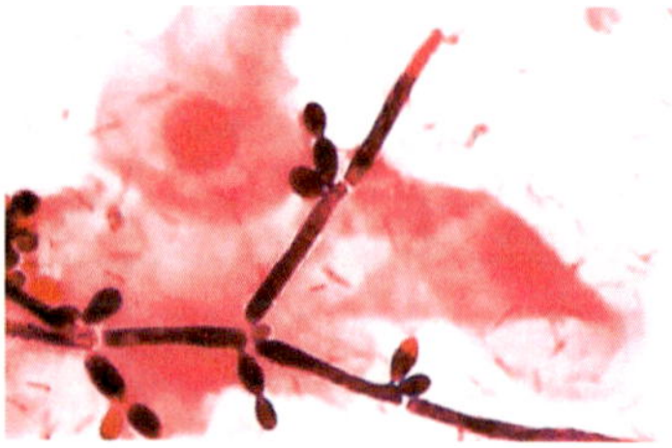

Page No. 88

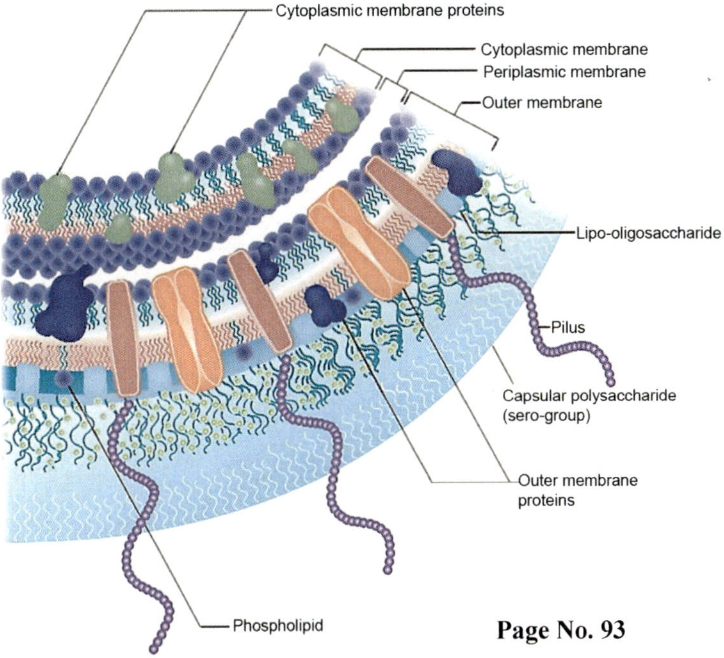

Page No. 93

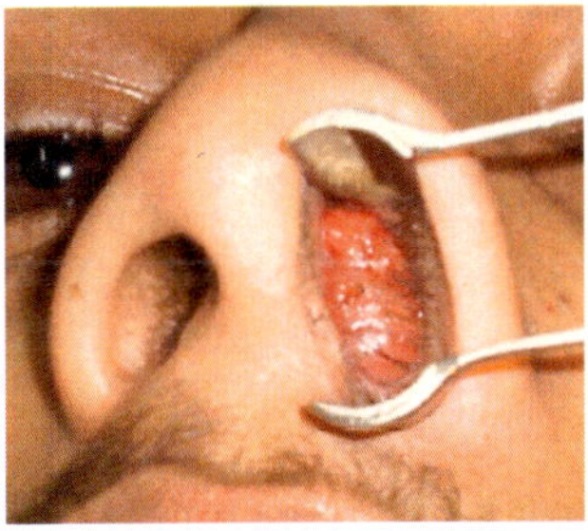

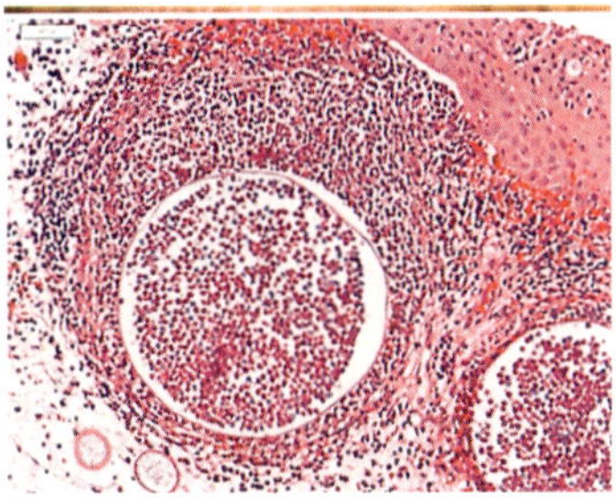

Page No. 100

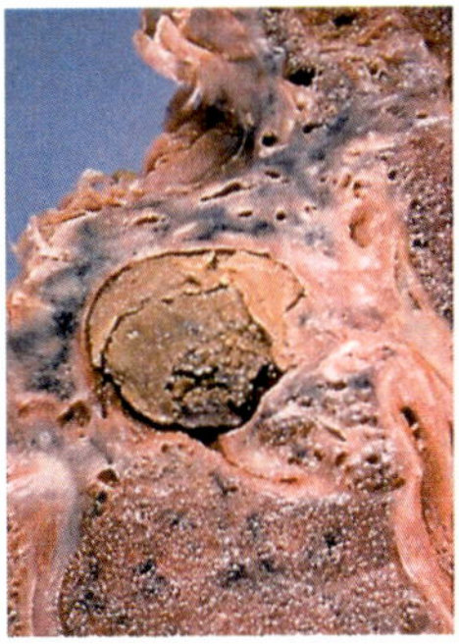

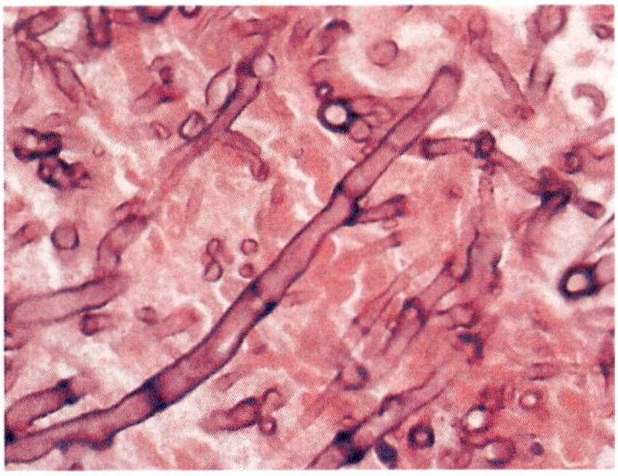

Page No. 105

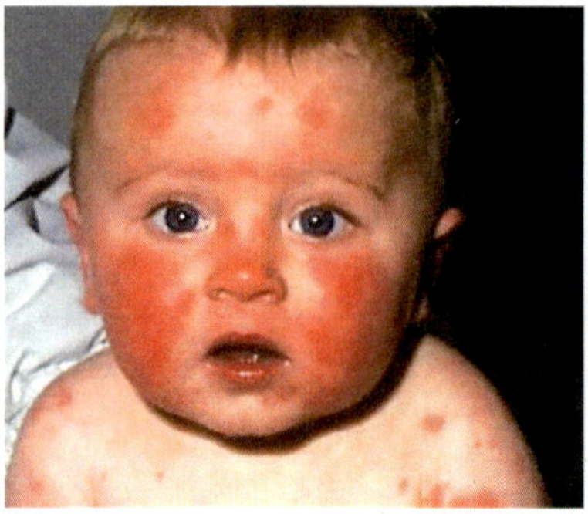

Page No. 103

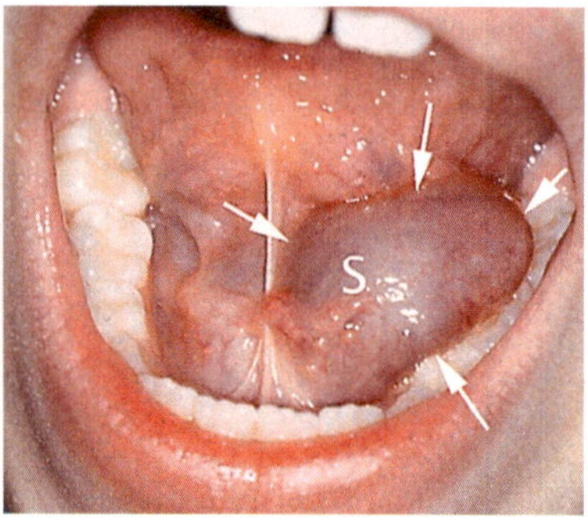

Page No. 207

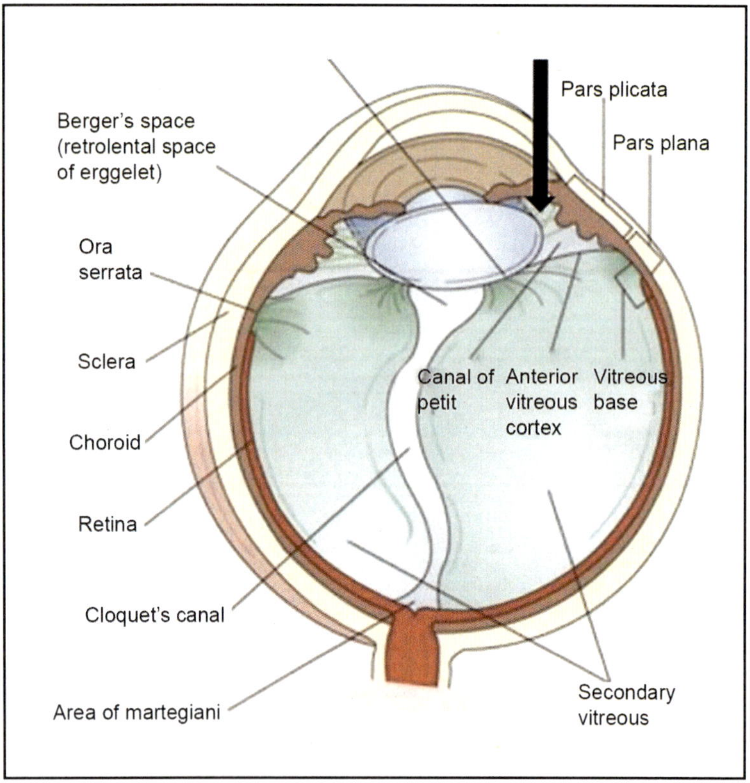

Page No. 176

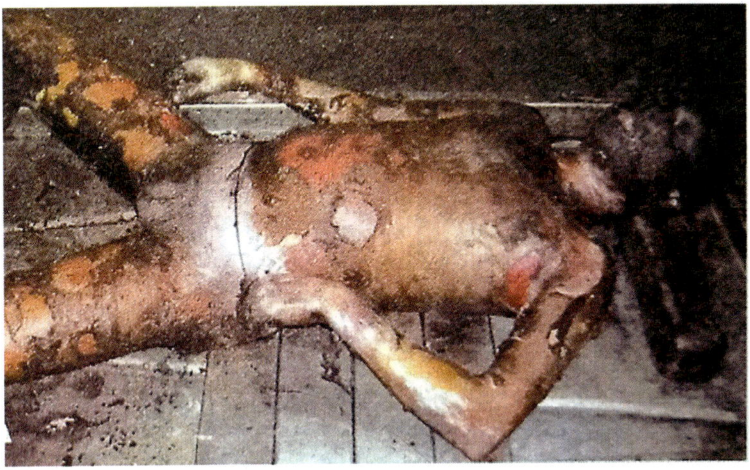

Page No. 145

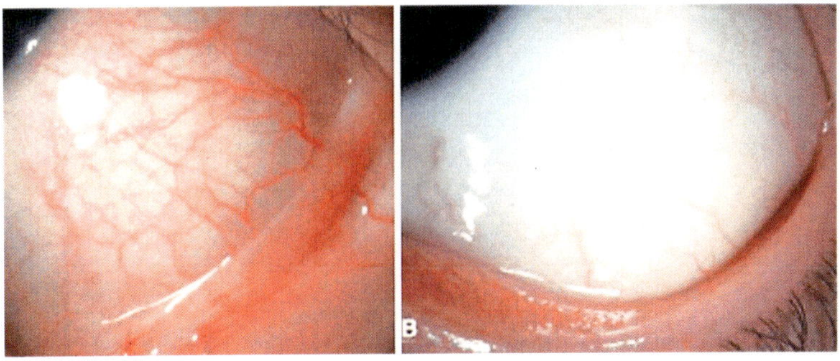

Page No. 178

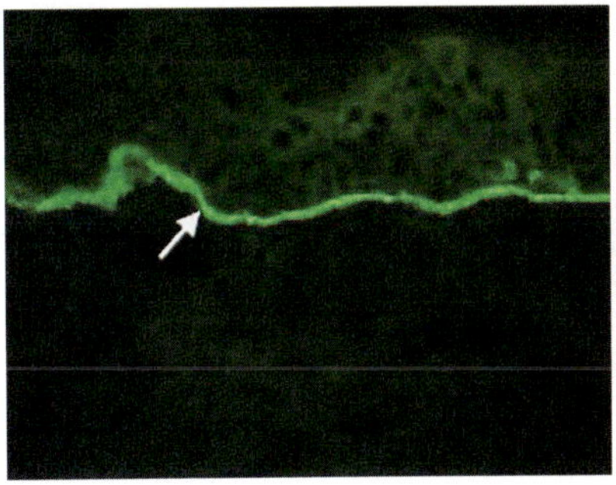

Page No. 261

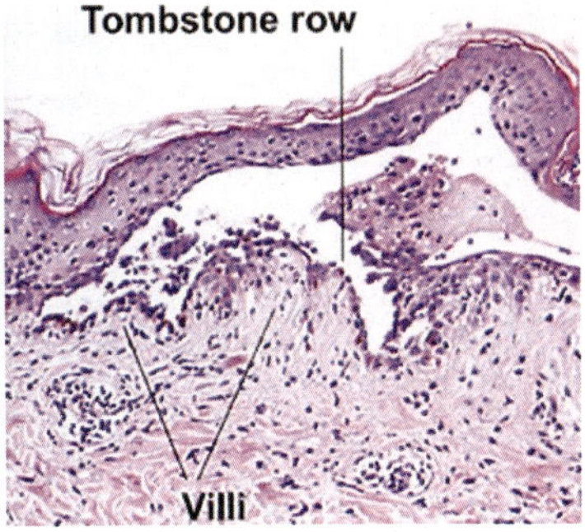

Page No. 267

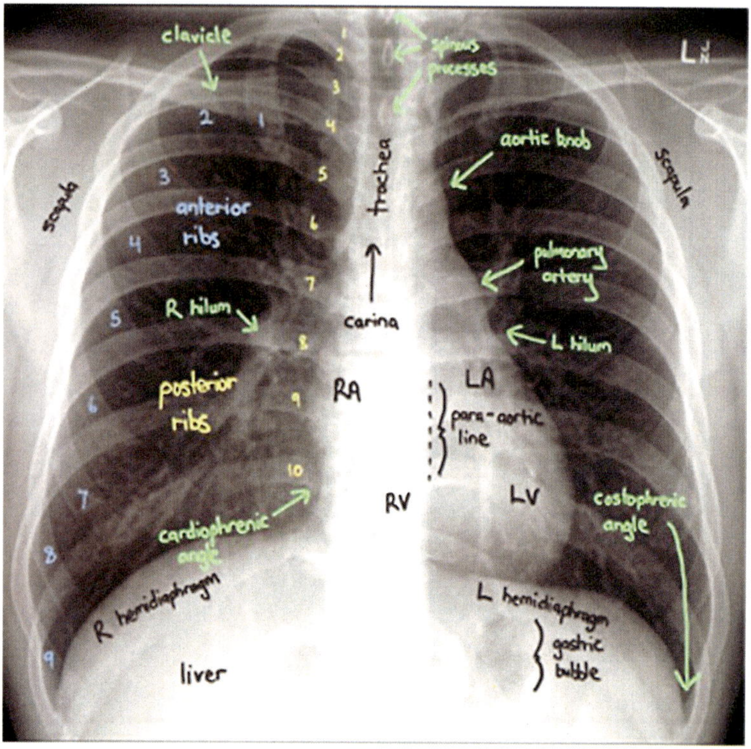

Page No. 294

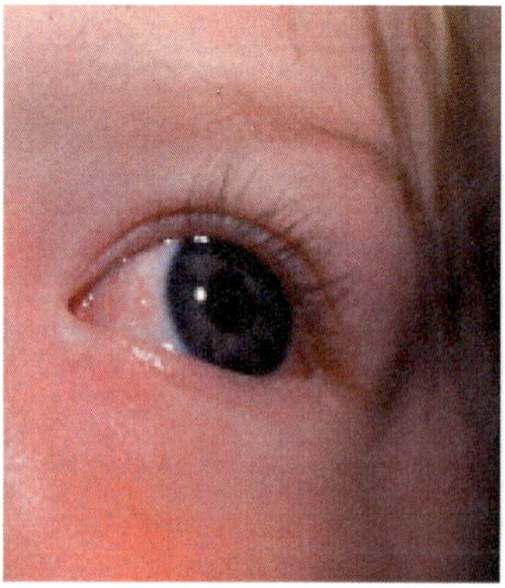

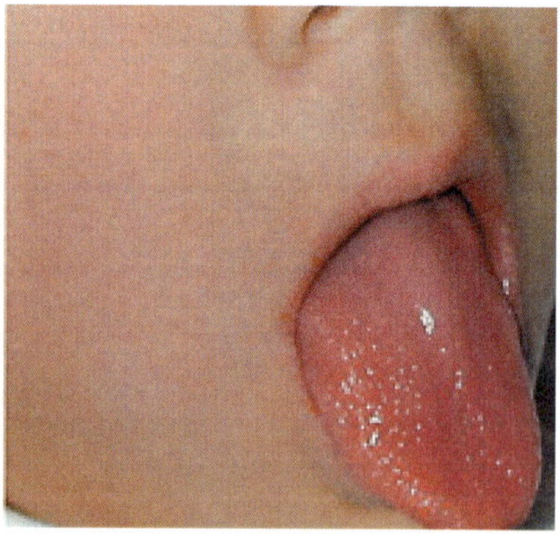

Page No. 301

ANATOMY

1. Match the following labels with the positions of the appendix:

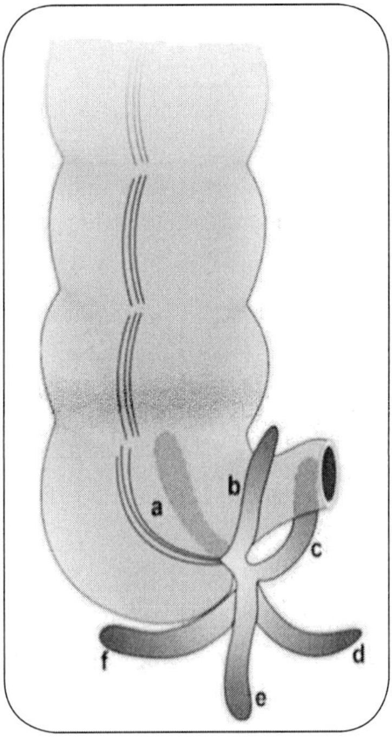

Label	*Position of the appendix*
a	1. Pre-ileal
b	2. Post-ileal
c	3. Retrocaecal
d	4. Pelvic
e	5. Paracaecal
f	6. Subcaecal

Lead – Choose the best answer from the codes given below:

A. a-3, b-1, c-2, d-4, e-6, f-5
B. a-3, b-4, c-1, d-5, e-2, f-6
C. a-5, b-2, c-3, d-4, e-1, f-6
D. a-5, b-6, c-3, d-2, e-1, f-4

Let's discuss the labels:

Label	*Position*	*Remarks*
a	Retrocaecal	• In about **60%** of individuals appendix lies behind the caecum, in the retrocaecal recess of the peritoneal cavity where part of it may lie behind the lower end of the ascending colon.
b	Pre-ileal	• The appendix may be in front of the terminal ileum.
c	Post-ileal	• The appendix may be behind the terminal ileum.
d	Pelvic	• In about **30%** individuals, the appendix extends downwards and medially into the true pelvis. • In this case, the appendix crosses the right external iliac artery. • In the female, it may lie close to the right ovary and uterine tube.
e	Subcaecal and Paracolic	• The appendix may be inferior to the caecum and the tip ascends to the side of the caecum.
f	Paracaecal	• Appendix lying alongside the lateral border of caecum.

2. Which of the following are the actions of the muscle shown in the image?

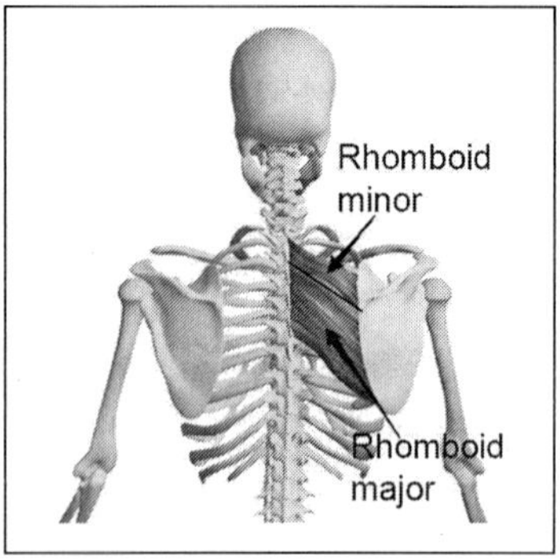

I. Retracts the scapula

II. Elevates the scapula

III. Rotates the scapula so that glenoid cavity face upwards

IV. Rotates the scapula so that glenoid cavity face downwards

Lead – Choose the best answer from the codes given below:

A. I and II
B. I and III
C. I and IV
D. II and III

Key points about movements of scapula:

- ***Retraction*** *means entire scapula slides backwards over the chest wall.*
- ***Elevation*** *means the entire scapula moves upwards (as in shrugging of shoulders).*
- *In forward (or lateral) rotation, the inferior angle of the scapula passes forwards and somewhat laterally. Simultaneously, the superior angle and the acromion pass backwards and medially. The glenoid cavity comes to face* ***upwards****. This movement takes place during abduction of the arm, and is essential in raising the arm above the head.*
- *In backward (or medial) rotation, the inferior angle of the scapula passes backwards and somewhat medially. Simultaneously, the superior angle and the acromion passes forwards and laterally. The glenoid cavity comes to face* ***downwards****.*

Let's discuss the options:

Option	*Statement*	*Remarks*
I	Retracts the scapula.	• True statement. • Retraction of the scapula is carried out by Rhomboideus major and Rhomboideus minor.
II	Elevates the scapula.	• False statement. • Elevation of scapula is done by Levator scapulae.
III	Rotates the scapula so that glenoid cavity face upwards.	• False statement. • This movement is carried by Trapezius and Serratus anterior.

Contd.

IV	Rotates the scapula so that glenoid cavity face downwards.	• True statement. • This movement is carried out by Rhomboideus major, Rhomboideus minor and Levator scapulae.

Coming back to the question:

- *The movements of retraction and rotation of the scapula (so that the glenoid cavity faces downwards) are brought about by rhomboideus major and rhomboideus minor muscles.*

3. In the floor of fourth ventricle, the lateral most nuclear column is:

A. GSA
B. SSA
C. SVE
D. SVA

Key points about nuclear columns:

- *Each half of the floor of the fourth ventricle is divided into a medial part and a lateral part by the* ***sulcus limitans****.*
- *Efferent nuclei lie in the medial part (called the basal lamina) and afferent nuclei in the lateral part (called the alar lamina).*
- *Within each category (for example, visceral efferents, somatic afferents etc.), the* ***general*** *nucleus lies nearer the sulcus limitans than the special nucleus.*
- *In each part (medial or lateral),* ***visceral*** *nuclei lie nearer to the sulcus limitans than somatic nuclei.*
- *So general visceral efferent and general visceral afferent nuclei lie nearer to the sulcus limitans.*
- *Thus, in proceeding laterally from the midline, the sequence of nuclear column is as follows:*
    - o *Somatic efferent: This column is not subdivided into general and special parts.*
    - o *Special visceral (or branchial) efferent.*
    - o *General visceral efferent.*
    - o *General visceral afferent.*
    - o *Special visceral afferent.*
    - o *General somatic afferent.*
    - o *Special somatic afferent.*

Nuclear columns in basal and alar laminae:

No.	*Nuclear columns of basal lamina*	*Nuclear columns of alar lamina*
1	• Somatic efferent.	• General visceral afferent.
2	• Special visceral efferent.	• Special visceral afferent.
3	• General visceral efferent.	• General somatic afferent.
4		• Special Somatic Afferent.

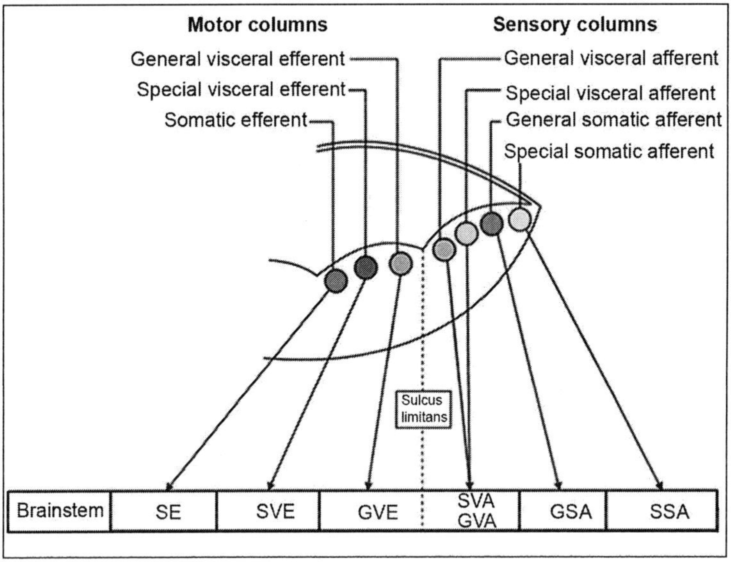

Coming back to the question:

- *Special Somatic Afferent is the lateral most nuclear column in the floor of fourth ventricle.*

4. Match the following:

Nerves	*Actions*
1. Facial nerve	**A. Shrugging of shoulder**
2. Mandibular nerve	**B. Chewing movements**
3. Spinal accessory nerve	**C. Taste sensations from anterior two-third of the tongue**
4. Glossopharyngeal nerve	**D. Sensory nerve supply from the face**
	E. Motor supply to stylopharyngeus

Lead – Choose the best answer from the codes given below:

A. 1-B, 2-A, 3-E, 4-C
B. 1-C, 2-B, 3-A, 4-E
C. 1-A, 2-B, 3-C, 4-E
D. 1-E, 2-A, 3-B, 4-D

Let's discuss the options:

Option	*Statement*	*Remarks*
1	Facial nerve	• Facial nerve gives origin to chorda tympani nerve, which is of considerable importance as it carries fibres of taste from the ***anterior*** two-thirds of the tongue and secretomotor fibres to the submandibular and sublingual glands. • Facial nerve supplies muscles of facial expression. • It passes through internal acoustic meatus and stylomastoid foramen.
2	Mandibular nerve	• Mandibular nerve is one of the branches of trigeminal nerve. • Mandibular nerve gives origin (from main trunk) to nerve to medial pterygoid, which supplies the **same** muscle (muscle of mastication).
3	Spinal accessory nerve	• Spinal part of the accessory nerve supplies sternocleidomastoid and the trapezius muscle. • Trapezius muscle is **tested** by shrugging of the shoulder.
4	Glosso-pharyngeal nerve	• Glossopharyngeal nerve winds round the stylopharyngeus muscle and it supplies it (this is the ***only*** motor branch of the glossopharyngeal nerve). • It carries proprioception from pharynx, larynx, palate and Eustachian tube. • It carries taste sensation from posterior one-third of tongue. • It provides parasympathetic supply to parotid. • It passes through jugular foramen.

Coming back to the question:

Nerves	*Actions*
1. Facial nerve	*C. Taste sensations from anterior two-third of the tongue*
2. Mandibular nerve	*B. Chewing movements*
3. Spinal accessory nerve	*A. Shrugging of shoulder*
4. Glossopharyngeal nerve	*E. Motor supply to stylopharyngeus*

5. Involvement of which artery lead to Lateral medullary syndrome?

A. Anterior spinal artery
B. Posterior inferior cerebellar artery
C. Middle cerebral artery
D. Anterior cerebral artery

Let's discuss the options:

Option	*Statement*	*Remarks*
a	Anterior spinal artery	• Occlusion of ASA produces **medial** medullary syndrome. • Ventral and medial part of medulla is damaged. • Involvement of **corticospinal** fibres (pyramids) leads to contralateral hemiplegia. • Damage to the **hypoglossal** nucleus leads to ipsilateral (lower motor neuron type of) paralysis of muscles of the tongue. • Involvement of the medial **lemniscus** leads to the loss of sensation of fine touch, sense of movement and sense of position.
b	Posterior inferior cerebellar artery	• Occlusion of PICA produces **lateral** medullary syndrome. • Damage to the lateral **spinothalamic** tract leads to contralateral loss of sensations of pain and temperature.

Contd.

		• Damage to the spinal nucleus and tract of the **trigeminal** nerve leads to loss of sensations of pain and temperature over the region supplied by the trigeminal nerve. • Damage to the nucleus **ambiguus** leads to difficulty in swallowing (dysphagia) and in speech (dysarthria). • Damage to the cerebellum and to the inferior cerebellar **peduncle** causes loss of equilibrium (ataxia) and giddiness. • Involvement of descending **autonomic** fibres leads to Horner's syndrome.
c	Middle cerebral artery	• Occlusion of MCA causes hemiplegia and loss of sensations on the opposite half of the body. The face and arms are **most** affected. Foot and leg **spared**. • Aphasia (by involvement of Broca's and Wernicke's area, especially if the thrombosis is in the left hemisphere in a right-handed person). • Homonymous hemianopia on opposite side (by involvement of optic radiation). • Hearing may be affected, but this may be compensated by opposite hemisphere.
d	Anterior cerebral artery	• Occlusion of ACA causes paralysis (or weakness) of muscles of the leg and foot of the opposite side (by involvement of the upper part of the motor area). • Loss (or dulling) of sensations from the leg and foot of the opposite side (by involvement of the upper part of the sensory area). • Sense of stereognosis is impaired (by involvement of parietal lobe). • **Personality** changes (by involvement of frontal lobe).

Coming back to the question:

- *Involvement of the posterior inferior cerebellar artery leads to lateral medullary syndrome.*

6. All of the following muscles are supplied by superior gluteal nerve EXCEPT:

A. Gluteus medius
B. Gluteus minimus
C. Piriformis
D. Tensor fascia lata

Let's discuss the options:

Option	*Statement*	*Remarks*
a, b	Gluteus medius Gluteus minimus	• Both are supplied by **superior** gluteal nerve (L5, S1). • Action is also common for both muscles. • Both muscles are **abductors** of the thigh. • The minimus and anterior fibres of medius can act as flexors and medial rotators. • Posterior fibres of the medius act as extensors and lateral rotators of thigh. • When the femur is fixed (as in standing), the medius and minimus pull their own side of the pelvis downward (by rotating it over the head of the femur). The opposite side of the pelvis is raised.
c	Piriformis	• It is supplied by **direct branches** from nerves (L5, S1, S2). • Act as lateral rotator of femur; abductor of flexed thigh.
d	Tensor fascia lata	• It is supplied by **superior** gluteal nerve (L4, L5, S1). • Helps to maintain erect posture. It stabilizes the pelvis on head of femur and the femur on the tibia. • Helps to extend the leg. • Helps in medial rotation of thigh. • May abduct the thigh.

Coming back to the question:

- *Piriformis is **NOT** supplied by superior gluteal nerve. It is supplied by direct branches from nerves (L5-S2).*

7. All of the following are relations of third part of duodenum EXCEPT:

A. Loops of jejunum
B. Root of mesentery
C. Superior mesenteric vessels
D. Gallbladder

Relations of third part of duodenum:

Anterior relations	*Posterior relations*
• Crossed by mesentery and superior mesenteric vessels. • Covered by transverse mesocolon, and sometimes by transverse colon, and/or • Loops of jejunum.	• Right psoas major. • Inferior vena cava. • Abdominal aorta. • Right ureter. • Right testicular or ovarian vessels. • Inferior vena cava and aorta separate it from vertebra L3.

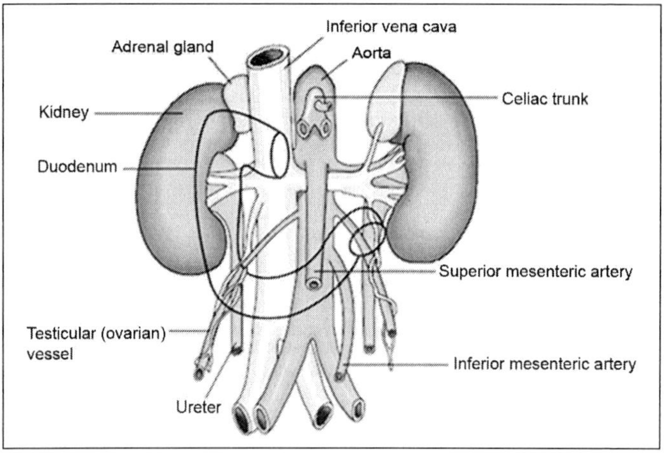

Coming back to the question:

- *Gallbladder is not related to the third part of duodenum.*

8. Location of SRY gene:

A. Short arm of chromosome X
B. Long arm of chromosome X

C. Short arm of chromosome Y

D. Long arm of chromosome Y

Key points about SRY gene:

- *SRY gene stands for **S**ex determining **R**egion of **Y** chromosome.*
- *It is present on **S**hort a**R**m of chromosome **Y.***
- *This gene produces a protein (testis-determining factor), that promotes the development of a testis.*
- *The primitive sex cords proliferate into the medulla to form the testicular cords.*
- *Some of those cells differentiate into Sertoli cells, whilst the remainder become incorporated into seminiferous tubules.*

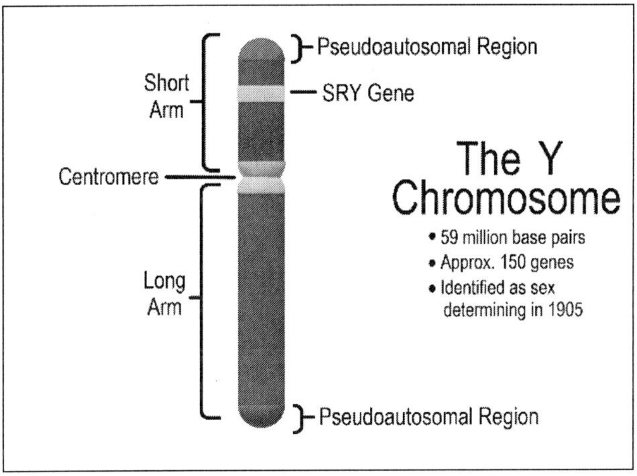

Coming back to the question:

- *SRY gene is located on the short arm of chromosome Y.*

PHYSIOLOGY

1. Which of the following is a true statement regarding the cells which are rich in smooth endoplasmic reticulum?

A. Concerned with protein synthesis
B. Concerned with steroid synthesis
C. Concerned with degradation of macromolecules
D. Concerned with production of energy

Let's discuss the options:

Option	*Statement*	*Remarks*
a	Concerned with protein synthesis	• Rough endoplasmic reticulum is concerned with synthesis (and folding) of proteins. • Rough endoplasmic reticulum is also known as granular endoplasmic reticulum because its surface is studded with **ribosomes**.
b	Concerned with steroid synthesis	• Smooth endoplasmic reticulum is concerned with steroid (non-protein) synthesis. • Smooth endoplasmic reticulum is the endoplasmic reticulum with smooth appearance. • Also known as agranular reticulum. • It is formed mainly by many interconnected tubules. • So it is also called **tubular** endoplasmic reticulum.
c	Concerned with degradation of macromolecules	• Lysosomes are digestive organelles of the cell. • Also known as '**suicidal** bag of the cell', because the interior of the lysosomes are always acidic. In the process of destroying the substrate, lysosomes are destroyed along with them.

Contd.

d	Concerned with production of energy	• Mitochondria produces ATP. • Involved in the synthesis of energyrich compound **ATP** by oxidative phosphorylation. • Also known as the powerhouse of the cell.

Coming back to the question:

- *Cells which are rich in smooth endoplasmic reticulum are concerned with steroid (non-protein) synthesis.*

2. Which of the following is the correct statement regarding excitation-contraction coupling mechanism of skeletal muscle?

A. Opening of voltage gated calcium channels is a prerequisite for contraction

B. Calcium is released from mitochondria

C. Extracellular calcium does not play any role

D. Calcium is not needed at all

Key points about excitation-contraction coupling/ECC:

- *It is the process that occur in between the excitation (electrical event) and contraction (mechanical event) of the muscle.*
- *This process involves series of activities, which are responsible for the contraction of the excited muscle.*
- *Stages of ECC:*
    - o *When a muscle is excited (stimulated) by the impulses passing through motor nerve and neuromuscular junction, action potential/AP is generated in the muscle fibre.*
    - o *This AP spread over the sarcolemma and also into the muscle fibre through the 'T' tubules.*
    - o *The 'T' tubules are responsible for the rapid spread of AP into the muscle fibre.*
    - o *When the AP reaches the cisternae of tubules, these cisternae are excited.*
    - o *Now the calcium ions stored in the cisternae are **released** into the sarcoplasm. Extracellular calcium does **not** play any role here.*

- *The calcium ions from the sarcoplasm move towards the actin filaments to produce the contraction.*
- *Thus the calcium ion forms the link or coupling material between the excitation and the contraction of muscle.*
- *Hence, the calcium ions are said to form the* ***basis*** *of excitation-contraction coupling.*

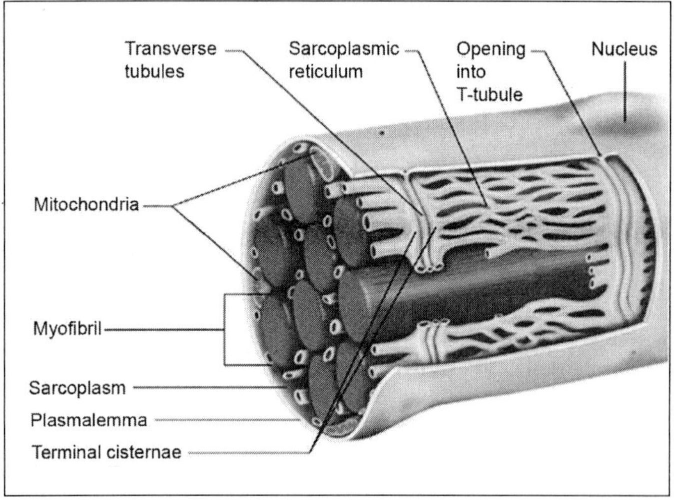

Let's discuss the options:

Option	*Statement*	*Remarks*
a	Opening of voltage gated calcium channels is a prerequisite for contraction in skeletal muscle	• False statement. • Voltage gated calcium channels are present in cardiac muscle and **not** in skeletal muscle. So they have nothing to do with contraction of skeletal muscle.
b	Calcium is released from mitochondria	• False statement. • Calcium released during excitation-contraction coupling comes from cisterns of T-tubules and **not** from mitochondria.

Contd.

c	Extracellular calcium does not play any role	• **True** statement. • Calcium released comes from cisterns of T-tubules. • When the AP reaches the cisternae of tubules, these cisternae are excited. • Now the calcium ions stored in the **cisternae** are released into the sarcoplasm. • Extracellular calcium does not play any role here.
d	Calcium is not needed at all	• False statement. • ECC is the process that occur in between the excitation (electrical event) and contraction (mechanical event) of the muscle. • Hence, the calcium ions are said to form the **basis** of excitation-contraction coupling.

Coming back to the question:

- *Extracellular calcium does not play any role in excitation contraction coupling. The calcium stored in the cisternae is the main source of calcium needed for ECC.*

3. Match the following:

Hormone	*Cells of secretion*
1. Gastrin	**A. S-cells of upper small intestine**
2. Secretin	**B. M-cells**
3. Motilin	**C. I-cells**
4. Cholecystokinin	**D. G-cells of antrum**

Lead – Choose the best answer from the codes given below:

A. 1-B, 2-A, 3-D, 4-C
B. 1-C, 2-B, 3-A, 4-D
C. 1-A, 2-B, 3-C, 4-D
D. 1-D, 2-A, 3-B, 4-C

Let's discuss the options:

Option	*Statement*	*Remarks*
1	Gastrin	• Gastrin is secreted by the **G** cells which are present in the pyloric glands of the stomach. • Small amount of gastrin is also secreted in mucosa of upper small intestine. • Three forms – G34, G17 and G14 gastrin. • G17 is the principal form. • Acts via CCK-B receptor. • Stimuli that **increase** gastrin secretion: Peptides, Amino acids, Epinephrine, Distension. • Stimuli that **decrease** gastrin secretion: Acid, Somatostatin, Secretin. • **Action**: Stimulation of gastric acid and pepsin secretion; stimulation of the growth of mucosa of GIT (trophic action).
2	Secretin	• Secretin is produced by **S** cells of mucous membrane in duodenum and jejunum. • It was the first hormone identified (by Bayliss and Staring). • It **increases** the secretion of bicarbonate by the duct cells of the pancreas and biliary tract (watery, alkaline juice). • Stimuli that **increases** release of secretin: Acid; Products of protein digestion.
3	Motilin	• Motilin is secreted by **Mo** cells, which are present in stomach and intestine. • It is also believed to be secreted by enterochromaffin cells of intestine. • Contracts smooth muscle in the stomach and intestines in between meal.

Contd.

4	Cholecystokinin	• It is secreted by **I** cells in duodenal and jejunal mucosa. • Also found in nerves in the distal ileum, colon and brain. • Acts via CCK-A receptor. • **Functions** in gut: Stimulation of pancreatic enzyme secretion; contraction of gallbladder; Relaxation of sphincter of Oddi. • Other actions: Augments the action of secretin; inhibits gastric emptying. • **Stimuli** that increases CCK secretion: Peptides and amino acids; Fatty acids (>10 C atoms).

Coming back to the question:

Hormone	***Cells of secretion***
1. Gastrin	*D. G-cells of antrum*
2. Secretin	*A. S-cells of upper small intestine*
3. Motilin	*B. M-cells*
4. Cholecystokinin	*C. I-cells*

4. The following graph has 2 curves. A is normal and B is some type of hypoxia. B curve depicts which type of hypoxia?

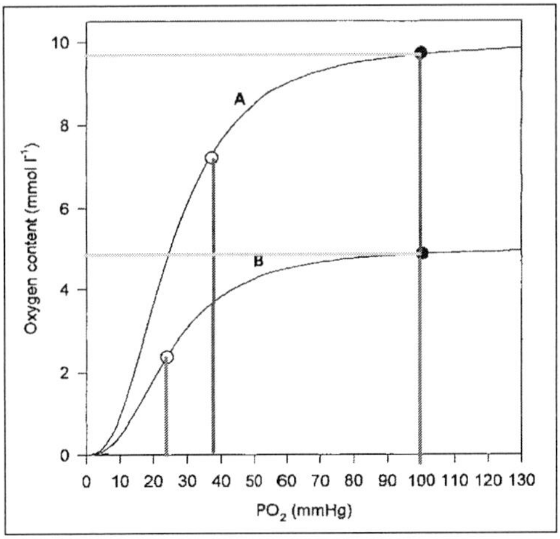

A. Hypoxic hypoxia
B. Anemic hypoxia
C. Stagnant hypoxia
D. Histotoxic hypoxia

Let's discuss the graph given in the question:

- *X-axis shows pO_2.*
- *Y-axis shows oxygen* ***content*** *(Y-axis in oxygen-haemoglobin dissociation curve represents percentage* ***saturation*** *of haemoglobin).*
- *A curve is normal and B curve is abnormal.*
- *Black circles denote arterial blood pO_2.*
- *White circles denote venous pO_2.*
- *Blue vertical line shows the pO_2 of arterial and venous blood respectively in normal state (curve A).*
- *Red vertical line shows the pO_2 of arterial and venous blood respectively in some hypoxic state (curve B).*
- *Pink horizontal line denotes the arterial oxygen content in normal state.*
- *Green horizontal line denotes the arterial oxygen content in some hypoxic state.*

Let's discuss the options:

Option	*Statement*	*Remarks*
a	Hypoxic hypoxia	• **pO_2** in arterial blood: **Reduced.** • O_2 carrying capacity of blood: Normal. • Velocity of blood flow: Normal. • Utilization of O_2 by tissues: Normal.
b	Anemic hypoxia	• **pO_2** in arterial blood: **Normal.** • O_2 carrying capacity/**content** of blood: **Reduced.** • Velocity of blood flow: Normal. • Utilization of O_2 by tissues: Normal.
c	Stagnant hypoxia	• pO_2 in arterial blood: Normal. • O_2 carrying capacity of blood: Normal. • **Velocity** of blood flow: **Reduced.** • Utilization of O_2 by tissues: Normal.

Contd.

d	Histotoxic hypoxia	• pO_2 in arterial blood: Normal. • O_2 carrying capacity of blood: Normal. • Velocity of blood flow: Normal. • **Utilization** of O_2 by tissues: **Reduced**.

Coming back to the question:

- *Findings of the abnormal curve B, which are consistent with the diagnosis of **anemic** hypoxia (can be correlated from the table):*
    - o ***pO_2** in arterial blood in both the curves A and B is **same** (blue and red vertical lines coinciding).*
    - o *O_2 carrying capacity/**O_2 content** of blood is **reduced** in curve B (big gap between pink and green horizontal lines).*

5. Relaxation pressure/airway pressure is zero at which of the following lung volume?

A. Inspiratory capacity
B. Total lung capacity
C. Residual volume
D. Functional residual capacity

Key points about Pressure-Volume curves of lung, chest wall and lung-chest wall combined:

- *Lung volume **Above** the FRC, the relaxation pressure/airway pressure is positive because the elastic recoil of the lung (inward) is greater than the outward elastic recoil of the chest wall. Collapsing forces dominate.*
- ***At** rest, lung volume is at the Functional Residual Capacity (the circled point in the graph shown below). Relaxation pressure is **0**. It is an equilibrium position.*
- *Lung volume **Below** the FRC, the relaxation pressure is negative because the recoil of the chest walls (outward) is greater than the recoil of the lung (inward). Expanding forces dominate.*

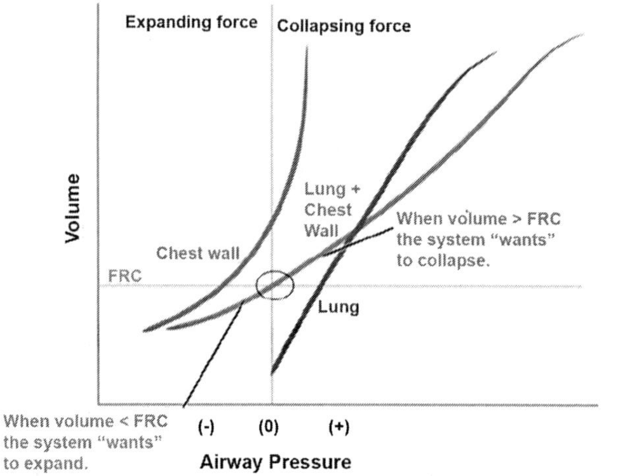

Functional Residual Capacity = Volume of air in lungs after tidal expiration (RV+ ERV). At this volume, the pulmonary system is in equilibrium because the collapsing force of the lungs is equal to the expanding force of the chest wall.

Let's discuss the options:

Option	*Statement*	*Remarks*
a	Inspiratory capacity	• Inspiratory capacity is the maximum volume of air that is inspired after normal expiration (end expiratory position). • It includes tidal volume and inspiratory reserve volume. • 3,800 mL.
b	Total lung capacity	• TLC is the volume of air present in lungs after a deep (maximal) inspiration. • It includes all the volumes. • 6,000 mL.
c	Residual volume	• RV is the volume of air remaining in lungs even after forced expiration. • Normally, lungs cannot be emptied completely even by forceful expiration. • It is significant as it helps to aerate the blood in between breathing and during expiration. • 1,200 mL.

Contd.

d	Functional residual capacity	• FRC is the volume of air remaining in the lungs after normal expiration (after normal tidal expiration). • FRC includes expiratory reserve volume and residual volume. • 2,200 mL. • At FRC, the system is relaxed meaning that the inward recoil of lung is balanced by the outward expansion of the chest wall (equilibrium point). • It is for this reason, FRC is also known as '**relaxation** volume' or 'equilibrium volume'.

Coming back to the question:

- *Relaxation pressure/airway pressure is zero at Functional residual capacity.*

6. Blood pressure changes in radial artery were measured during Valsalva manoeuvre/VM. Initially, increase in BP is due to which of the following reason:

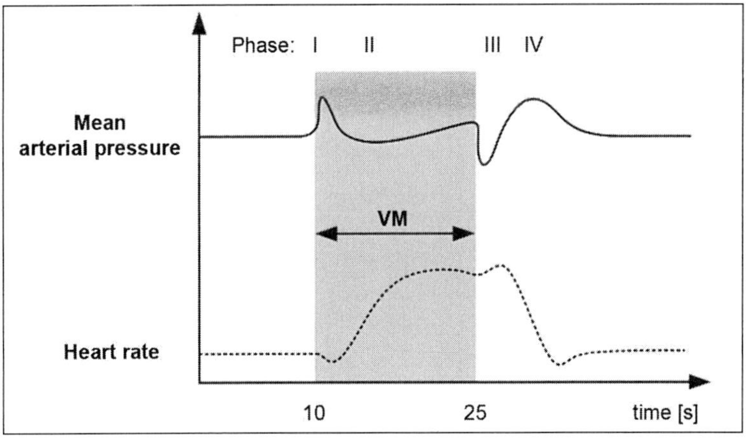

A. Increase in aortic pressure
B. Increase in left ventricular pressure
C. Increase in left ventricular volume
D. Increased venous return

Key points about Valsalva manoeuvre:

- *It is the forced expiratory effort with closed glottis.*
- *It is performed by attempting to exhale forcibly, while keeping the mouth and nose closed.*
- *It* ***provides*** *information about the components of baroreflex through variations in BP and heart rate.*
- *Phases of Valsalva manoeuvre and its effect on BP:*
    - *Phase I:*
        - *Onset of straining.*
        - *There is short rise in BP due to sudden increase in intrathoracic pressure, which increases* ***aortic*** *pressure too.*
    - *Phase II:*
        - *Maintain strain.*
        - *There is decrease in BP due to decrease in venous return.*
    - *Phase III:*
        - *Release stress.*
        - *There is decrease in arterial pressure due to sudden release and decrease in intrathoracic pressure.*
    - *Phase IV:*
        - *Overshoot.*
        - *There is increase in BP due to increase venous return.*

Let's discuss the options:

Option	***Statement***	***Remarks***
a	Increase in aortic pressure	• **True** statement. • In phase I of Valsalva manoeuvre/VM, there is initial short rise in BP due to sudden increase in intrathoracic pressure which increases aortic pressure.
b	Increase in left ventricular pressure	• False statement. • In phase I of Valsalva manoeuvre, there is initial short rise in BP due to sudden increase in intrathoracic pressure which increases aortic pressure (**not** because of increase in left ventricular pressure).

Contd.

c	Increase in left ventricular volume	• False statement. • Increased venous return → increase in left ventricular volume → an increase in BP, mainly in phase **IV** of Valsalva manoeuvre (**not** in phase I).
d	Increased venous return	• False statement. • Increased venous return causes an increase in BP, mainly in phase **IV** of Valsalva manoeuvre (**not** in phase I).

Coming back to the question:

- *Increase in BP during initial phase of Valsalva manoeuvre is because of raised intrathoracic pressure, which increases aortic pressure.*

7. What is the correct order of arrangement of structures in sarcomere, going from outside to inside?

A. Z line – A band – H zone – M line
B. A band – Z line – H zone – M line
C. M line – A band – Z line – H zone
D. H zone – A band – Z line – M line

Key points about sarcomere:

- *Each sarcomere extends between two '**Z**' lines of myofibril.*
- *Each myofibril consists of an alternate dark '**A**' band and light 'I' band.*
- *A band is the length of myosin filament.*
- *I band is the space between the tip of two myosin filaments of adjacent sarcomeres.*
- *In the middle of the 'A' band, there is a light area called '**H**' zone.*
- *'H' zone is the space between the two actin filaments of the same sarcomere.*
- *In the middle of the 'H' zone lies the middle part of myosin filament. This is called '**M**' line.*
- *M line is formed by myosin binding proteins.*

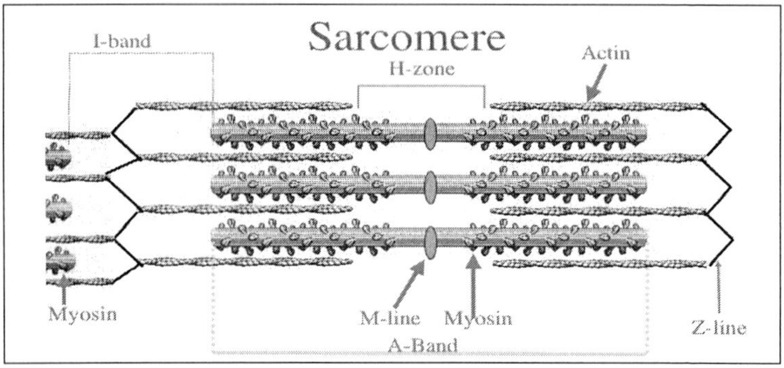

Coming back to the question:

- *The correct order of structures in sarcomere (going from outside to inside) is: Z line – A band – H zone – M line.*

8. All of the following vessels shows Windkessel effect EXCEPT:

A. Aorta
B. Common carotid artery
C. Radial artery
D. Subclavian artery

Key points about Windkessel effect:

- *It is the recoiling effect of blood vessels that converts the pulsatile flow of blood into a continuous flow.*
- *Blood vessels showing the Windkessel effect are known as Windkessel vessels.*
- *During systole, velocity of blood flow reaches maximum, because of the force created by contraction of the heart. Therefore, the maximum volume of blood is pumped into the aorta.*
- *During diastole, this force is absent and the volume of blood entering the aorta is zero. Thus, the blood flow into the aorta is not continuous. This type of blood flow is known as **pulsatile** flow.*
- *However, the flow of blood, through the other blood vessels is continuous.*
- *It is because of the behavioural pattern of aorta and to a little extent, the behavioural pattern of larger arteries.*
- *During systole, the aorta is completely dilated and during diastole, it recoils.*
- *The **elastic** recoiling of this vessel creates the continuous momentum of blood. So the pulsatile flow of blood is converted into a **continuous** flow.*

- *This effect was named as Windkessel effect by Otto Frank, in 1889. Windkessel is a German word used for elastic reservoir.*
- *Thus, the Windkessel effect plays an important role in maintaining the continuous flow of blood through the circulatory tree by acting as a* ***second*** *pump, the first pump being the heart.*
- *Aorta and its large branches are considered as Windkessel vessels (elastic arteries).*

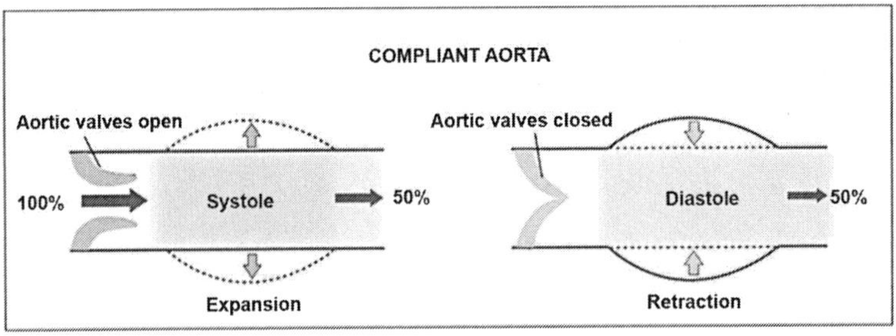

Let's discuss the options:

Option	*Statement*	*Remarks*
a	Aorta	• Elastic artery (Windkessel vessel).
b	Common carotid artery	• Elastic artery (Windkessel vessel).
c	Radial artery	• Muscular artery (**not** a Windkessel vessel).
d	Subclavian artery	• Elastic artery (Windkessel vessel).

Coming back to the question:

- *Radial artery is* ***NOT*** *an example of windkessel vessel, as it is a muscular artery (not an elastic artery).*

9. Which of the following is a JAK-STAT pathway regulated hormone?

A. Leptin B. Aldosterone
C. Calcitonin D. Vasopressin

Key points about receptors for hormones:

- *Hormone influence cellular function by acting through the receptors present in the cell.*
- *Water soluble hormones like protein and peptide hormones can't cross the cell membrane. So, they act through receptors present*

*outside the cell in cell **membrane** receptors; extracellular receptors).*

- *Cell membrane receptors are of **4** types:*
  - o *G-protein coupled receptor/GPCR:*
    - ♦ *Coupling of hormone-receptor complexes by G-protein activates **3** second messenger systems like Adenylyl cyclase – cAMP system, Inositol triphosphate (IP_3) – Diacylglycerol (DAG) system or Guanylyl cyclase – cGMP system.*
  - o *Receptor tyrosine kinase.*
  - o *Cytokine receptor family (JAK/STAT).*
  - o *Receptor serine/threonine kinase.*
- *Lipid soluble hormones like steroid hormones and vitamin derivatives can cross the cell membrane. They act through the receptor present in cell nucleus (**nuclear** receptors; intracellular receptors).*

Let's discuss the options:

Option	*Statement*	*Remarks*
a	Leptin	• Leptin acts by binding to the cytokine receptor and interacts with an important intracellular kinase called Janus kinases (JAK). • Janus kinase (JAK) phosphorylates members of signal transduction and activators of transcription (STAT) family – **JAK/STAT** pathway.
b	Aldosterone	• It acts through **nuclear** receptor. • Aldosterone acts through messenger RNA (mRNA) mechanism. • Since aldosterone is lipid soluble, it diffuses readily into cytoplasm of the tubular epithelial cells through the lipid bilayer of the cell membrane. • In the cytoplasm, aldosterone binds with the specific receptor protein. • Aldosterone-receptor complex diffuses into the nucleus where it binds to deoxyribonucleic acid and causes formation of mRNA.

Contd.

c	Calcitonin	• Acts through adenylyl cyclase-**cAMP** second messenger system.
d	Vasopressin	• Vasopressin (**V**$_1$ receptor) acts through IP_3-DAG-calcium second messenger system. • Vasopressin (**V**$_2$ receptor) acts through adenylyl cyclase-cAMP second messenger system.

Coming back to the question:

- *Leptin is a JAK-STAT pathway regulated hormone.*

BIOCHEMISTRY

1. All of the following amino acids are used for the synthesis of hormones EXCEPT:

A. Glycine
B. Tryptophan
C. Phenylalanine
D. Tyrosine

Let's discuss the options:

Option	***Statement***	***Remarks***
a	Glycine	• Glycine may be used for the biosynthesis of: o Creatine, Creatine phosphate and Creatinine. o Heme. o Purine nucleotides; and o Glutathione. • **No** hormones are produced directly or indirectly.
b	Tryptophan	• Substances produced from tryptophan are: o Alanine (glucogenic). o Acetoacetyl CoA (ketogenic). o Niacin and NAD^+. o Serotonin. o Melatonin. o Hydroxy-Indole-Acetic Acid (excretory product); and o Indican (excretory product).
c	Phenylalanine	• Phenylalanine is converted into Tyrosine (by phenylalanine hydroxylase enzyme), which is used for synthesis of hormones. • So **indirectly**, phenylalanine is needed for synthesis of hormones.

Contd.

d	Tyrosine	• Important specialized products from tyrosine are: o Melanin. o Catecholamines (epinephrine); and o Thyroxine.

Coming back to the question:

- *Glycine is **NOT** needed for synthesis of any hormone.*

2. A young boy was a known case of type I diabetes mellitus. He presented with unconsciousness with emanation of peculiar smell from the nostrils. His urine was subjected to some test and the result is shown below. Which test is being performed?

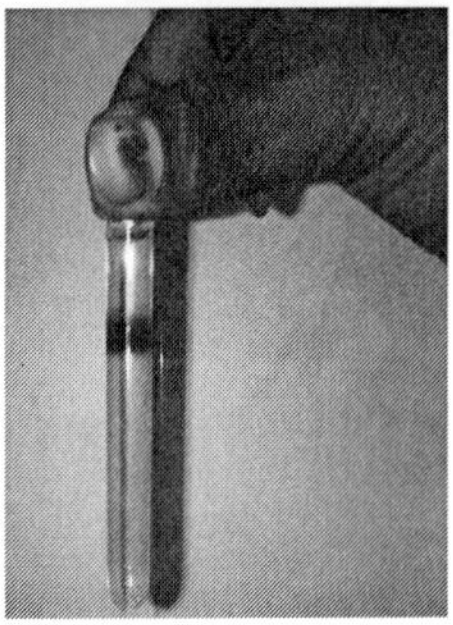

A. Fouchet's test
B. Biuret reaction
C. Rothera's test
D. Benedict's reaction

Clinical presentation in the question is indicative of diabetic ketoacidosis.

Key points about Diabetic ketoacidosis/DKA:

- *Ketosis is **more** common in type I diabetes mellitus.*
- *Normally the blood level of ketone bodies is **less** than 1 mg/dL and **only** traces are excreted in urine (not detectable by usual tests).*
- *But when the rate of synthesis **exceeds** the ability of extrahepatic tissues to utilize them, there will be accumulation of ketone bodies in the blood.*
- *This leads to ketonemia, excretion in urine (ketonuria) and **smell** of acetone in breath.*
- *All these three together constitute the condition known as ketosis.*
- *American Diabetes Association/ADA **criteria** for DKA include:*
    - o *Serum glucose >250 mg/dL.*

- o *Serum anion gap >10 mEq/L.*
- o *Bicarbonate <18 mEq/L.*
- o *Serum pH <7.30; and*
- o *Presence of ketosis.*

- *Management guidelines:*
    - o *Parenteral administration of Insulin to control diabetes.*
    - o *Insulin promotes transfer of extracellular potassium back to intracellular compartment, causing dangerous hypokalemia, which should be promptly corrected.*
    - o *Intravenous bicarbonate to correct the acidosis.*
    - o *Correction of water imbalance by normal saline.*

Let's discuss the options:

Option	***Statement***	***Remarks***
a	Fouchet's test	• Fouchet's test is done to test **bile** pigments. • Urine is heated with barium sulfate, which adsorbs bilirubin. • Ferric chloride oxidizes bilirubin to produce a **green** color.
b	Biuret reaction	• Biuret reaction is a color reaction of amino acids and **proteins.** • Cupric ions in an alkaline medium form a **violet** color with peptide bond nitrogen. • This needs a minimum of two peptide bonds, and so individual amino acids and dipeptides will not answer this test. • This reaction can be used for quantitative estimation also. • The name is derived from the compound biuret, a condensation product of two urea molecules, which also gives a positive color test.

Contd.

c	Rothera's test	• The presence of ketosis can be established by the detection of **ketone** bodies in the urine by Rothera's test. • Saturate 5 mL of urine with solid ammonium sulfate. • Add a few drops of freshly prepared sodium nitroprusside followed by 2 mL of liquor ammonia along the sides of the test tube. • Development of a purple **ring** indicates the presence of ketone bodies in urine. • The clinical presentation in the questions is indicative of diabetic ketoacidosis.
d	Benedict's reaction	• Benedict's reagent is very commonly employed to detect the presence of glucose in the urine (glycosuria). • It is a standard laboratory test employed for follow-up of diabetes mellitus. • Benedict's reagent contains sodium carbonate, copper sulfate and sodium citrate. • In alkaline medium, sugars form enediol, cupric ions are reduced, correspondingly sugar is oxidized. • Glucose is a **reducing** sugar. • Any sugar with free aldehyde/keto group will reduce the Benedict's reagent. • Therefore, this is **not** specific for glucose.

Coming back to the question:

- *Rothera's test is done to detect ketone bodies in urine, which is indicated by formation of a purple ring.*

3. Liver cannot utilise ketone bodies because of lack of the enzyme:

A. Thioesterase
B. Thiolase
C. Thiophorase
D. Thiokinase

Key points about ketolysis:

- *The ketone bodies are formed in the liver; but they are utilized by extrahepatic tissues.*
- *The heart muscle and renal cortex* ***prefer*** *the ketone bodies to glucose as fuel.*
- *Tissues like skeletal muscle and brain can* ***also*** *utilize the ketone bodies as alternate sources of energy, if glucose is not available.*
- *Acetoacetate is activated to acetoacetyl CoA by* ***thiophorase*** *enzyme.*
- *Then acetoacetyl CoA enters the beta oxidation pathway to produce energy.*
- *Almost all tissues and cell types can use ketone bodies as fuel, with the* ***exception*** *of liver and RBC.*
- *The placenta can also use ketone body as fuel.*
- *Intestinal mucosal cells, brain and adipocytes use ketone bodies.*
- *Skeletal muscles, heart, liver, etc. primarily utilize fatty acids during starvation.*

Let's discuss the options:

Option	***Statement***	***Remarks***
a	Thioesterase	• Thioesterase enzyme is needed for **de novo** synthesis of fatty acids. • Thioesterase/TE or deacylase activity releases palmitate from the multienzyme complex. • The end point is palmitic acid (16C) in liver and adipose tissue.
b	Thiolase	• Thiolase is an important enzyme needed for **beta**-oxidation of fatty acids. • It mediates step 4 of beta-oxidation of fatty acids, by converting beta-keto fatty acyl CoA into fatty acyl CoA (2 carbon atoms less) + Acetyl CoA.

Contd.

c	Thiophorase	• Thiophorase is an important enzyme in **ketolysis**. • The ketone bodies are formed in the liver; but they are utilized only by extrahepatic tissues. • The heart muscle and renal cortex **prefer** the ketone bodies to glucose as fuel. • Tissues like skeletal muscle and brain can **also** utilize the ketone bodies as alternate sources of energy, if glucose is not available. • Acetoacetate is activated to acetoacetyl CoA by **thiophorase** enzyme. • Then acetoacetyl CoA enters the beta oxidation pathway to produce energy. • Almost all tissues and cell types can use ketone bodies as fuel, with the **exception** of liver and RBC.
d	Thiokinase	• Fifth step in **Kreb's** cycle involves a substrate level phosphorylation whereby a high energy phosphate is generated from the energy trapped in the thioester bond of succinyl CoA. • This reaction is mediated by succinate thiokinase.

Coming back to the question:

- *Although liver produces ketone bodies, but it itself **cannot** utilize those ketone bodies as it lacks thiophorase enzyme.*

4. What will be the sequence of new mRNA if the template DNA strand is having sequence is 5' CGTTATTTACTA 3'?

A. 5' GCAATAAATGAT 3'
B. 5' GCAAUAAAUGAU 3'
C. 5' UAGUAAAUAACG 3'
D. 5' CGUUAUUUACUA 3'

Key points about transcription:

- *Both DNA strands can serve as template for transcription but for a given gene, only one strand act as a template.*
- *So each time one is template strand and other is non-template strand, depending on the gene.*
- ***Template** strand:*
    - o *The template strand is one of the strand of DNA which serve as a template for the synthesis of mRNA, for a particular gene.*
    - o *Now when the template strand is transcribed, then new mRNA sequence is complimentary to it (there will be U in RNA, which pairs with A in DNA).*
    - o *The template strand is therefore known as anti-sense/non-coding or minus strand.*
- ***Non-template** strand:*
    - o *The sequence of other non-template DNA is same like mRNA (but there is U in place of T), so therefore non-template strand is also known as coding strand.*
    - o *Direction of new mRNA is same like the non-template strand so the non-template strand is also known as **sense** strand or plus strand.*

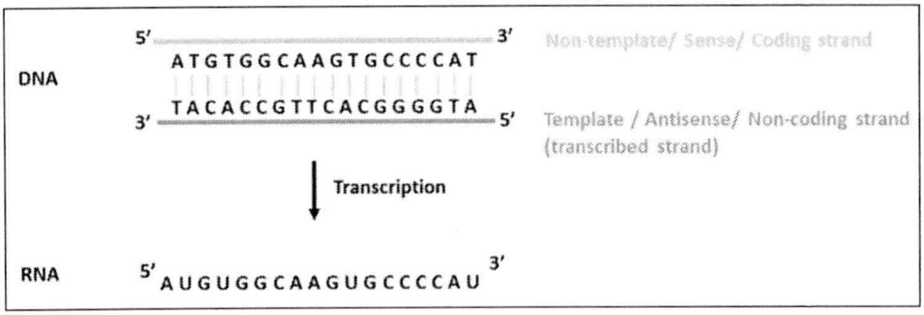

How to solve such question?

- *Write the **template** strand (of DNA), which is usually given in 5' to 3' direction in questions.*
- ***Derive** the non-template strand/sense strand (of DNA) by A-T and G-C pairing formula, and it is written in 3' to 5' direction.*
- *Now **reverse** the sequence of bases to get it into 5' to 3' direction. If the template strand is given in 3' to 5' direction, then **no** need to reverse as the non-template/sense strand will be derived in 5' to 3' direction.*
- *For mRNA sequence, **replace** all T's with U.*

Coming back to the question:

- *The DNA* ***template*** *strand given in the question is* **5' CGTTATTTACTA 3'.**
- *So let us* ***derive*** *the non-template/sense strand following C-G and A-T base pairing rule, it will come out to be* **3' GCAATAAATGAT 5'.**
- *Here 3' is on the left side and 5' is on the right side, now we have to arrange this so that 5' is on the left side and 3' is on the right side (****reverse*** *the sequence).*
- *So, we get* **5' TAGTAAATAACG 3'.**
- *Now for RNA,* ***replace*** *all T's to U.*
- *So answer comes out to be* **5' UAGUAAAUAACG 3'.**

5. Deficiency of which of the following vitamin can result in excretion of Xanthurenic acid in urine?

A. Vitamin B_1 B. Vitamin B_2
C. Vitamin B_6 D. Vitamin B_{12}

Let's discuss the options:

Option	*Statement*	*Remarks*
a	Vitamin B_1	• In thiamine deficiency, blood thiamine is reduced, but pyruvate, alpha ketoglutarate and lactate are increased. • Erythrocyte **transketolase** activity is reduced; this is the earliest manifestation seen even before clinical disturbances.
b	Vitamin B_2	• Active moiety: FAD (Flavin adenine dinucleotide), FMN (Flavin mono-nucleotide). • Sources: Milk, egg, liver, fish etc. • Endogenously synthesized by bacterial flora. • Main biochemical reaction: Oxidation – reduction reactions. • Biochemical assessment of deficiency: Erythrocyte **glutathione** reductase activity is reduced.

Contd.

		• Deficiency: Riboflavinosis (oro-oculo-genital syndrome).
c	Vitamin B_6	• Active form of pyridoxine is pyridoxal phosphate (PLP). • PLP acts as coenzyme for many reactions in amino acid metabolism. • PLP is required for the synthesis of niacin from tryptophan. • One vitamin is needed for synthesis of another vitamin. • 3-hydroxy kynurenine → 3-hydroxy-anthranilic acid (enzyme kynureninase). • Kynureninase is a PLP dependent enzyme. • Hence is vitamin B_6 deficiency, niacin production is less. • Moreover, kynureneine cannot be converted further, which is metabolized to **xanthurenic** acid and is excreted through urine.
d	Vitamin B_{12}	• Active moiety: Methylcobalamin. • Sources: Milk, curd, cheese, egg, liver, meat, fish (**only** found in animal sources). • Main biochemical role: Synthesis of methionine, isomerization of methyl **malonyl** CoA. • Deficiency: Megaloblastic anemia, Sub-acute combined degeneration, Demye-lination, Pernicious anemia.

Coming back to the question:

- *Xathurenic aciduria is seen in deficiency of vitamin B_6.*

6. All of the following statements are true for collagen EXCEPT:

A. It is a fibrillary protein

B. Cross-linkage formation needs copper and vitamin C

C. Proline and hydroxylproline are present

D. Phenylalanine is the most abundant amino acid

Key points about collagen:

- *Collagen is the most abundant protein in mammals and is the main fibrous component of skin, bone, tendon, cartilage and teeth.*
- *Collagen forms a superhelical cable where 3 polypeptide chains are wound around itself.*
- *Each polypeptide chain of collagen has about 1000 amino acid residues.*
- *The amino acid composition of collagen is quite unique.*
- *About 33% of the amino acids is* ***glycine****, that is, every third residue is glycine.*
- *The repetitive amino acid sequence may be represented as Gly – X – Y – Gly – X – Y; where X and Y are other amino acids, most commonly proline and hydroxyproline.*
- *The only amino acid that can fit into the triple stranded helix is glycine.*
- *Replacement of the central glycine by mutations can lead to brittle bone disease.*
- *The triple helix of collagen is stabilized by the steric repulsion of the rings of* ***hydroxyproline*** *and also by the hydrogen bonds between them.*
- *The hydroxylation of* ***proline*** *and lysine residues of collagen is a post-translational modification taking place intracellularly.*
- *Prolyl hydroxylase and lysyl hydroxylase are both dioxygenases using molecular oxygen.*
- *The enzyme contains ferrous ions at its active site and require a reducing agent like* ***ascorbic*** *acid to preserve the iron in the reduced ferrous state.*
- *So vitamin C deficiency leads to poor hydroxylation.*
- *In vitamin C deficiency, failure of hydroxylation of proline/lysine leads to reduced hydrogen bonding and consequent weakness of collagen.*
- *The collagen fibers are strengthened by covalent crosslinks between lysine and hydroxyl-lysine residues.*

- *The crosslinks are formed by lysyl oxidase which converts these amino acids into aldehydes.*
- *Lysyl oxidase is a copper containing enzyme, the copper ion being located at its active site.*
- *In* ***copper*** *deficiency, reduced cross linking of collagen results.*

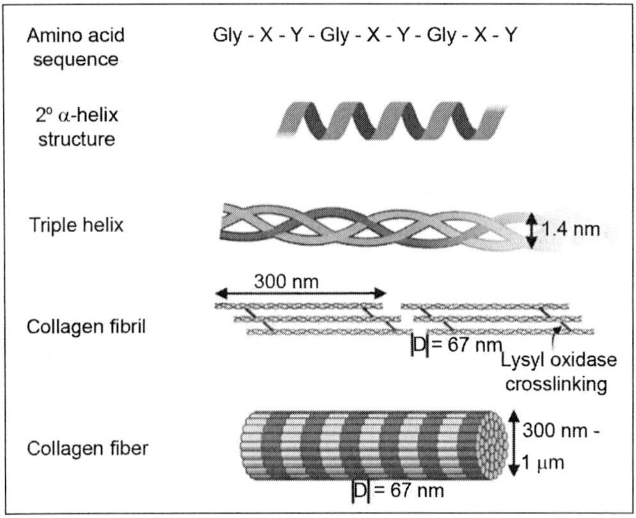

Coming back to the question:

- *Phenylalanine is* ***NOT*** *the abundant amino acid in collagen. The abundant amino acid in collagen is Glycine.*

7. Pompe's disease is because of deficiency of the enzyme:

A. Beta-glucosidase B. Phosphofructokinase
C. Muscle phosphorylase D. Alpha 1, 4 glucosidase

Let's discuss the options:

Option	*Statement*	*Remarks*
a	Beta-glucosidase	• Deficiency of Beta-glucosidase causes **Gaucher's** disease (lipid storage disease). • It is an inborn error of metabolism due to failure of degradation of glucocerebrosides.

Contd.

		• Glucocerebroside is the **accumulating** lipid. • 3 types: Adult, infantile and juvenile. • Hepatosplenomegaly. • Erosion of bone. • Moderate anemia.
b	Phosphofructokinase	• Deficiency of muscle Phosphofructokinase-1 (muscle, RBCs) causes **Tarui's** disease (Type VII glycogen storage disease). • Glycogen accumulates in muscles. • Exercise intolerance. • Hemolytic anemia.
c	Muscle glycogen phosphorylase	• Deficiency of muscle phosphorylase (skeletal muscle) causes **McArdle's** disease (Type V glycogen storage disease). • Exercise intolerance. • Accumulation of glycogen in muscles. • Myoglobinuria.
d	Alpha 1, 4 glucosidase	• Deficiency of Alpha 1, 4 glucosidase (Lysosomal maltase) causes **Pompe's** disease (glycogen storage disease II). • Accumulation of glycogen in lysosomes of liver, heart and muscle. • In infantile form, death occurs before 2 years. • Juvenile form presents with myopathy. • Adult form has muscular dystrophy like presentation.

Coming back to the question:

- *Pompe's disease occurs because of deficiency of the enzyme alpha 1, 4 glucosidase.*

8. True statement regarding thermic effect:

A. Equal for all the fuels
B. Highest for fats
C. Highest for proteins
D. Highest for carbohydrates

Key points about thermogenic effect of food:

- *Energy required to digest, absorb, transport and metabolize the food material is known as thermogenic effect of food.*
- *It is **maximum** for proteins, then carbohydrates and **least** for fats.*
- *Thermogenic effect of food is **also** known as the thermic effect of food or SDA (specific dynamic action) or DIT (diet induced thermogenesis).*
- *It leads to the production of heat in the body, e.g., in brown fat.*

Coming back to the question:

- *Thermic effect is highest for proteins.*

9. Barth syndrome usually presents with cardiac failure. In such cases, which of the following structures is deficient in inner mitochondrial membrane of heart muscles?

A. Plasmalogen
B. Lecitin
C. Cardiolipin
D. Lysolecithin

Let's discuss the options:

Option	*Statement*	*Remarks*
a	Plasmalogen	• These are phospholipids which have an aliphatic long chain alpha-beta unsaturated alcohol in ether linkage with the first hydroxyl group of glycerol. • The second OH group is esterified to a fatty acid. • The phosphoric acid is attached to choline or ethanolamine.

Contd.

		• The alcohols have about C12 to C18 chain length. • Plasmalogens are found in bio-membranes in brain and muscle.
b	Lecithin	• Also known as phoshatidylcholine. • This is a nitrogen containing phospholipid. It contains glycerol. • The alpha and beta positions are esterified with fatty acids. • Usually, the fatty acid attached to the beta-carbon, is a PUFA molecule. • The phosphoric acid is added to the third position, to form phosphatidic acid. • The phosphate group is esterified to the quaternary nitrogen base, choline. • Dipalmitoyl Lecithin is one of the main constituent of surfactant. • Low surfactant level can lead to respiratory distress syndrome. • The lecithin sphingomyelin (LS) ratio of amniotic fluid index of fetal maturity. A ratio of 2 indicates full lung maturity.
c	Cardiolipin	• It is formed by when two molecules of phosphatidic acid are linked with a molecule of glycerol (diphosphatidylglycerol). • It is the major lipid of **mitochondrial** membrane. • Commercially, it is extracted from myocardium. • Decreased cardiolipin level leads to mitochondrial dysfunction, and is accounted for heart failure, hypothyroidism and some type of myopathies (Barth syndrome).

Contd.

d	Lysolecithin	• Phospholipases are enzymes that hydrolyse phospholipids. Different phospholipases are involved in the hydrolysis of specific bonds in lecithin. • Phospholipase A2 acts on an intact lecithin molecule hydrolysing the fatty acid esterified to the beta (second) carbon atom. • The products are lysolecithin and fatty acid. • Lysolecithin is a detergent and hemolytic agent. • The enzyme is present in the venom of viper snakes. • The hemolysis and consequent renal failure seen in viper poisoning could be thus explained.

Coming back to the question:

- *Barth syndrome occurs because of deficiency of cardiolipin in inner mitochondrial membrane of heart muscles.*

10. Study the pedigree chart shown below and interpret the pattern of inheritance:

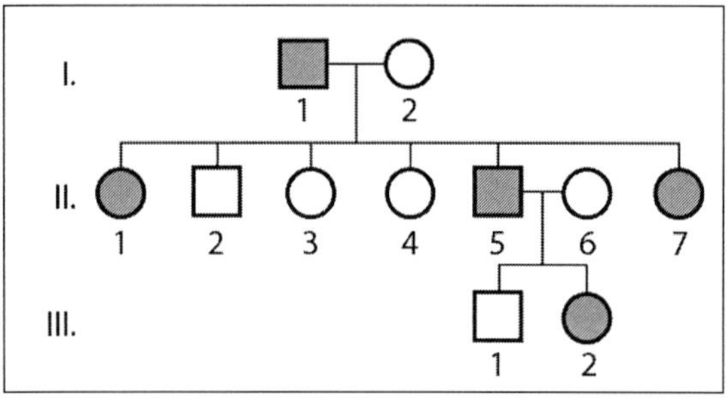

A. Autosomal dominant
B. Autosomal recessive
C. Incomplete penetrance
D. Pseudodominant inheritance

Let's discuss the options:

Option	*Statement*	*Remarks*
a	Autosomal dominant	• It is characterized by the phenotypic expression of the disease, even if one allele is abnormal or in heterozygous state. • Affected men (square) and women (circle) transmit the abnormality to their children. • When an affected heterozygote parent has a normal spouse, half **(50%)** of the progeny will have the disease. • The trait may be transmitted by either parent and can affect both male and female offsprings. • Every generation is affected.
b	Autosomal recessive	• Increased risk of transmission to siblings produced as a result of consanguineous marriages. • Occurs when both alleles at a given locus are mutated. • Disease is manifested only in homozygous state. • For example, in person suffering from sickle cell anemia, both the alleles for beta-globin have mutated. Hence, all beta, globin chains will be abnormal. He is homozygous for sickle cell disease/SCD. • In certain cases, the carrier state may be identified biochemically, then it is referred to as the trait of the disease. For example, in sickle cell trait, one beta-globin gene (allele) is normal, while the other one is abnormal (carrier state). Such individual is heterozygous to that character. Therefore, normal gene produces normal Hb and abnormal gene produces HbS. Thus inside the RBC, 50% of hemoglobin molecules are abnormal.

Contd.

		• When both the father and mother are carriers, one-quarter **(25%)** of siblings express the disease (both alleles abnormal), another one-quarter (25%) are normal, and half of the children are carriers. • If only one parent is carrier and the other is normal, then there will be no affected child, but 50% children are carriers. When an affected child is born, each subsequent child has a 25% chance of being affected. • Most of the inborn errors of metabolism are recessively transmitted.
c	Incomplete penetrance	• Incomplete penetrance describes when some people with a disease-causing mutation (change) in a gene develop the disease, while others don't. • For example, certain gene mutations cause cancer, but because of incomplete penetrance, not everyone who has the mutations, will develop cancer.
d	Pseudo-dominant inheritance	• Pseudodominant inheritance occurs when an individual with a known recessive disorder has a clinically unaffected partner, but then unexpectedly gives birth to children who are affected with the same recessive disorder as the affected parent. • Such disorders can be easily distinguished from classical dominant inheritance with molecular diagnosis and haplotype analysis.

Coming back to the question:

- *In given pedigree, in Generation I: Affected male (**1**) marries unaffected female (2).*
- *Generation II: They have six children:*
    - *Four daughters (1, 3, 4 and 7) out of which two were affected (**1** and 7).*
    - *Two sons (2 and 5), out of which one was affected (**5**).*

- *Generation III: Affected son (**5**) marries a normal female (6) and this couple have 2 children, out of which one was affected (**2**).*
- *So all the generations showed **50%** transmission, if only one parent was affected.*
- *Moreover, every generation was affected.*
- *So this pedigree is suggestive of autosomal dominant pattern of inheritance.*

PATHOLOGY

1. Which of the following statement is true for thymoma?

A. X-ray is the investigation of choice
B. Thymoma is the most common neoplasm of thymus
C. Thymoma can cause dysphagia
D. It is most commonly located in posterior mediastinum

Key points about thymoma:

- *Thymoma is the **most** common primary tumour present in the **antero**superior mediastinum.*
- *Thymoma remains asymptomatic in about half of the cases.*
- *Other patients have associated conditions like myasthenia gravis or local symptoms such as cough, dyspnoea and chest pain.*
- *Thymoma remains **asymptomatic** in about half of the case and may be accidentally discovered in X-rays.*
- *But CT scan is the first **choice** modality in differentiating thymoma from thymic lymphoid hyperplasia.*
- *On CT, thymomas usually present as sharply demarcated round or oval soft tissue masses in the anterior mediastinum compartment.*
- *This typical appearance is highly suggestive of the diagnosis.*

Coming back to the question:

- *Thymoma is most common neoplasm of thymus.*

2. Match the following:

Condition	*Feature*
1. Caplan syndrome	**A. Pleural effusion is seen without mediastinal shift**
2. Mesothelioma	**B. Initially described in coal workers**
3. Silicosis	**C. Involves lower lobe of lung predominantly**
4. Asbestosis	**D. Crazy paving pattern on HRCT scan**

Lead – Choose the best answer from the codes given below:

A. 1-B, 2-A, 3-D, 4-C
B. 1-C, 2-B, 3-A, 4-D
C. 1-A, 2-B, 3-C, 4-D
D. 1-C, 2-A, 3-B, 4-D

Let's discuss the options:

Option	*Statement*	*Remarks*
1	Caplan syndrome	• The development of rheumatoid arthritis in a few cases of **coal worker's** pneumoconiosis, silicosis or asbestosis is termed rheumatoid pneumoconiosis or Caplan's syndrome. • The lung lesions in Caplan's syndrome have immunological basis for their origin as evidenced by detection of rheumatoid factor and antinuclear antibodies.
2	Mesothelioma	• Mesothelioma is an uncommon tumour arising from mesothelial lining of serous cavities, most often in pleural cavity, and rarely in peritoneal cavity and pericardial sac. • Malignant or diffuse mesothelioma is significant in view of its recognised association with occupational exposure to asbestos (especially crocidolite) for a number of years, usually 20 to 40 years. • About 90% of malignant mesothelioma are asbestos-related. • Homozygous deletion of tumour suppressor gene CDKN2A/INK4a is common. • Thick, firm, white pleural tumour ensheathes the lung. • Clinical manifestations include chest pain, dyspnoea, pleural **effusion** and infections. • Prognosis is poor; 50% of patients die within one year of diagnosis.

Contd.

3	Silicosis	• It is caused by inhalation of silica. • Silica occurs in crystalline and amorphous forms. • Crystalline form (e.g., quartz) are more fibrogenic. • Form nodules in the upper zones of the lungs. • X-ray: Egg shell calcification in the lymph nodes. • High resolution CT (HRCT) scans may show the characteristic **crazy** paving appearance, caused by airway filling and interlobular septa thickening. • Silicosis is associated with increased susceptibility to tuberculosis and lung cancer.
4	Asbestosis	• The gross pulmonary fibrosis caused by asbestos exposure and histologic demonstration of asbestos bodies on asbestos fibres is known as asbestosis. • Grossly, the affected lungs are small and form with cartilage-like thickening of the pleura. • The sectioned fibres shows variable degree of pulmonary fibrosis, especially in the subpleural areas and in the **bases** of the lungs. • Asbestosis related disease include pleural plaques (most common manifestation of asbestos exposure), pleural effusions, parenchymal interstitial fibrosis (asbestosis), lung carcinoma, mesotheliomas (pleural and peritoneal) etc.

Coming back to the question:

Condition	*Feature*
1. Caplan syndrome	*B. Initially described in coal workers*
2. Mesothelioma	*A. Pleural effusion is seen without mediastinal shift*
3. Silicosis	*D. Crazy paving pattern on HRCT scan*
4. Asbestosis	*C. Involves lower lobe of lung predominantly*

3. Such a stain is used to study:

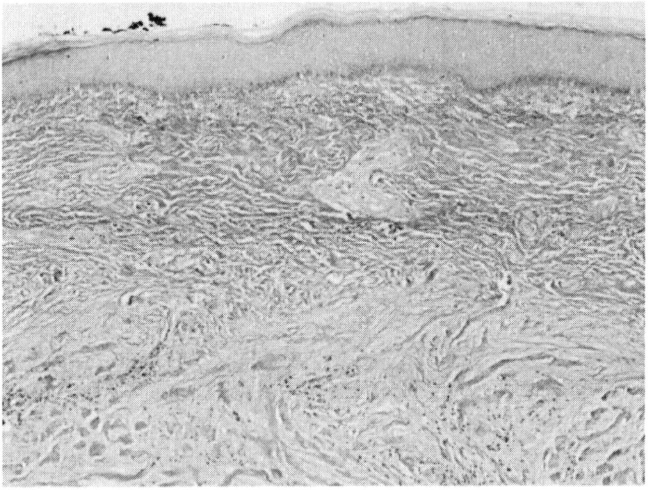

A. Amyloidosis
B. Collagen
C. Elastic fibres
D. Osteoid

Image shows Masson trichrome staining.

Key points about Masson trichrome stain:

- *It is a three-colour staining procedure.*
- *It is suited for distinguishing cells from surrounding connective tissue.*
- *Most recipes produce **red** keratin and muscle fibers, **blue**/green collagen and bone, light red/**pink** cytoplasm, and dark **brown**/black cell nuclei.*

Let's discuss the options:

Option	*Statement*	*Remarks*
a	Amyloidosis	• Stains used for diagnosing amyloid are Hematoxylin and Eosin/H and E stain, Methyl violet/Crystal violet stain, Congo red stain, Thioflavin-T/Thioflavin-S stain and immunohistochemistry.
b	Collagen	• Stain used for collagen are: H and E stain, Masson's trichrome stain and Van Gieson stain.
c	Elastic fibres	• Elastic fibers do not stain with the usual stains for collagen. • They can be demonstrated by staining with orcein, with aldehyde fuchsin, and by Verhoeff's method.
d	Osteoid	• Uncalcified osteoid appears eosinophilic in H and E stains and does not stain with Von Kossa reaction. • Mineralized osteoid is basophilic in appearance and stains black with Von Kossa reaction (a stain for calcium).

Coming back to the question:

- *Masson trichrome stain is used to stain collagen.*

4. Smudge cells were seen on a peripheral smear of a patient. Most appropriate next investigation in such a patient would be:

A. Complete blood count
B. Flow cytometry
C. Bone marrow biopsy
D. Cytogenetical studies

Clinical presentation is indicative of chronic lymphocytic leukaemia/ CLL.

Key points about CLL:

- *Median age at diagnosis: 60 years.*
- *Male : female ratio is 2 : 1.*
- *Morphological hallmark on microscopy are proliferation centers.*

- *Peripheral smear: Small round lymphocytes with scant cytoplasm and smudge cells.*
- ***Smudge**/Basket cells (degenerated forms) are present due to damaged nuclei of fragile malignant lymphocytes (blue arrow in the given image).*
- *Immunophenotype: Tumour cells are positive for CD19, CD20, CD23 and CD5.*
- *Associated with autoimmune hemolytic anemia.*

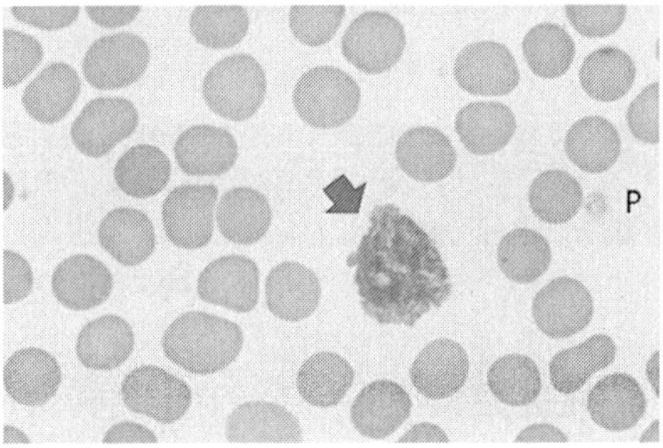

Let's discuss the options:

Option	*Statement*	*Remarks*
a	Complete blood count	• CBC show absolute lymphocytosis $>5\times10^9$/ L
b	Flow cytometry	• Peripheral blood flow cytometry is the **most** valuable test to confirm a diagnosis of CLL. • This test can determine that the cancer is CLL and not another form of leukaemia. • It confirms the presence of circulating clonal B-lymphocytes expressing CD5, CD19, CD20 (dim), CD23 and an absence of FMC-7 staining.
c	Bone marrow biopsy	• The typical findings of CLL on bone marrow examination are: Increased lymphocyte count (25-95%), reduced myeloid precursors and reduced erythroid precursors.

Contd.

d	Cytogenetical studies	• FISH. • Most common cytogenetic abnormality seen in CLL is trisomy 12 (seen in about 25% cases).

Coming back to the question:

- *In a patient, in whom smudge cells are seen on peripheral smear (clinical diagnosis: CLL), flow cytometry is the next appropriate investigation.*

5. Which of the following procedures are NOT used to detect DNA sequence?

I. Flow cytometry
II. Pyrosequencing
III. FISH
IV. PCR

Lead – Choose the best answer from the codes given below:

A. I and II
B. I and III
C. I, II and III
D. I, II, III and IV

Let's discuss the options:

Option	*Statement*	*Remarks*
I	Flow cytometry	• **False** statement. • Flow cytometry is a computerised technique by which the detailed characteristics of individual tumour cells are recognised and quantified and the data can be stored for subsequent comparison too. • Since, for flow cytometry, single cell suspensions are required to 'flow' through the 'cytometer', it can be employed on blood cells and their precursors in bone marrow aspirates and body fluids, and sometimes on fresh-frozen fixed tissue.

Contd.

		• The method employs either identification of cell surface antigen (e.g., in classification of leukaemias and lymphomas), or by the DNA content analysis (e.g., aneuploidy in various cancers).
II	Pyrosequencing	• **True** statement. • Pyrosequencing is a method of DNA **sequencing** that differs from Sanger sequencing, in that it relies on the detection of pyrophosphate release and the generation of light on nucleotide incorporation, rather than chain termination with deoxynucleotides.
III	FISH	• **False** statement. • In situ hybridization/ISH has gained popularity over other molecular biology methods because the DNA/mRNA of interest can be viewed in context of the tissue morphology. • When the probe is tagged with fluorescein, it can be seen under UV microscope; then it is called FISH (fluorescent in situ hybridization). • Examples of applications of ISH and FISH are: (a) assessment of gene rearrangements in leukaemia (b) diagnosis of B-cell lymphoma by demonstration of reduced light-chain mRNA (c) determination of amplification of HER2/neu in breast cancer and (d) diagnosis of various type of lymphoma.
IV	PCR	• **True** statement. • Polymerase chain reaction of an in vitro DNA amplification procedure in which multiple copies of a particular **sequence** of DNA can be produced within few hours.

Contd.

		• It is like Xerox machine for gene copying. • Applications of PCR: (a) detection of infectious diseases like AIDS, TB (b) detection of variations and mutations in genes like prenatal diagnosis of genetic disorders (c) DNA fingerprinting – can multiply small amounts of DNA found in blood samples, hair, semen and other body fluids.

Coming back to the question:

- *Pyrosequencing and PCR are the methods related to DNA sequence. Flow cytometry and FISH are not at all related to DNA sequencing.*

6. Which of the following is an anti-apoptotic gene?

A. BAX B. Bad

C. Mcl-1 D. BAK

Key points about apoptosis:

- *Also known as programmed cell death.*
- *Apoptotic cells break into fragments, known as apoptotic bodies.*
- *Plasma membrane of the apoptotic cell and bodies remain intact.*
- *Content of cell do not leak out, thus, it does not elicit any inflammatory response.*
- *Apoptosis results from the activation of enzymes known as caspases.*
- *Two phases:*
    - o *Initiation phase: Anti-apoptotic (growth promoter) proteins Bcl-2, Bcl-x are inhibited and pro-apoptotic proteins like BAX, BAK are activated (intrinsic/mitochondrial pathway).*
    - o *Execution phase: Activation of caspases 9, 8 and 10 in the initiation phase, results in activation of executioner caspases, i.e., caspase 3 and 6.*
- *Morphology:*
    - o *Cell shrinkage (as compared to cell swelling in other types of cell injury).*

- o *Chromatin condensation.*
- o *Formation of cytoplasmic blebs and apoptotic bodies.*
- o *Phagocytosis of apoptotic cells or cell bodies.*

Let's discuss the options:

Option	*Statement*	*Remarks*
a	BAX	• Pro-apoptotic protein.
b	Bad	• Pro-apoptotic protein.
c	Mcl-1	• Anti-apoptotic protein.
d	BAK	• Pro-apoptotic protein.

Coming back to the question:

- *Mcl-1 is an anti-apoptotic protein.*

7. Which of the following is the most common cause of hyper-coagulable state?

A. Deficiency of protein C and S
B. Mutation in Factor V Leiden
C. Deficiency of antithrombin III
D. Defects in fibrinolysis

Let's discuss the options:

Option	*Statement*	*Remarks*
a	Deficiency of protein-C and S	• Both these are autosomal dominant disorders having either reduced amount of protein C or S, or both, or their functional defect. • Clinically both are conditions associated with lifelong risk of thrombosis of deep leg veins.
b	Mutation in Factor V Leiden	• This is also an autosomal dominant disorder in which the mutation lies in replacement of arginine by glycine at position 506. • It is the **most** common cause of thrombophilia (hypercoagulable state).

Contd.

c	Deficiency of antithrombin III	• It is inherited as autosomal dominant disorder having less than 50% anti-thrombin III. • The condition is associated with recurrent episodes of venous thrombosis.
d	Defects in fibrinolysis	• These include a few **rare** inherited disorders such as dysfibrinogenaemia and plasminogen disorders.

Coming back to the question:

- *Mutation in factor V Leiden is the most common cause of hypercoagulable state.*

8. Which of the following changes are associated with necrosis?

I. Cell swelling

II. Ruptured cell membrane

III. Inflammation

IV. Physiological

Lead – Choose the best answer from the codes given below:

A. I and II
B. II and III
C. I, II and III
D. I, II, III and IV

Key points about necrosis:

- *It is the form of cell death in which there occurs denaturation of intracellular proteins and enzymatic digestion of injured cell.*
- *Plasma membrane damage results in leakage of protein contents outside the cell that elicits an inflammatory reaction.*
- *Morphology:*
  - o *Myelin figures: Large whorled phospholipid masses, derived from damaged cell membrane.*
  - o *Marked dilation of mitochondria with appearance of **large** amorphous densities.*
  - o *Nuclear changes like karyolysis, pyknosis and karyorrhexis.*
- *Patterns of necrosis:*
  - o *Coagulative necrosis: Due to ischaemia caused by obstruction in a vessel. It can be seen in all organs **except** the brain.*

- o *Liquefactive/Colliquative necrosis: Digestion of dead cells, results in transformation of tissue into a liquid viscous mass.* ***Most*** *commonly affects central nervous system.*
- o *Gangrenous necrosis: Represents coagulative pattern of necrosis. Seen in lower limb, that has lost its blood supply and has undergone necrosis.*
- o *Caseous necrosis: Cause cheese like necrosis. Microscopy shows amorphous granular debris with inflammatory cells and granuloma formation.*
- o *Fat necrosis: Seen in pancreas and peritoneum. Due to release of pancreatic lipases from pancreas in acute pancreatitis. Lipases split triglyceride esters within the fat cells, which combine with calcium to produce chalky-white areas (fat saponification).*
- o *Fibrinoid necrosis: Seen in immune reactions involving blood vessels. Vessel wall appears bright pink and amorphous on H and E stain, called fibrinoid (fibrin like).*

Let's discuss the options:

Option	***Statement***	***Remarks***
I	Cell swelling	• **True** statement. • Cell swelling is seen initially in necrosis.
II	Ruptured cell membrane	• **True** statement. • There is membrane disruption in necrosis.
III	Inflammation	• **True** statement. • Inflammation reaction is always present in necrosis.
IV	Physiological	• **False** statement. • Necrosis is **never** physiological. • It can be caused by various agents such as hypoxia, chemical and physical agents, microbial agents, immunological injury etc.

Coming back to the question:

- *In necrosis, there is an initial cell swelling, ruptured cell membrane, inflammatory reaction etc. but necrosis is not a physiological process.*

9. Identify the cell shown below:

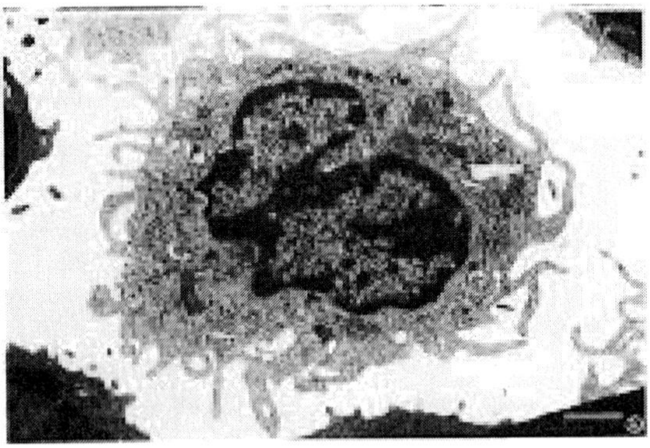

A. Sickle cell
B. Target cell
C. Gaucher's cell
D. Hairy cell

Let's discuss the options:

Option	*Statement*	*Remarks*
a	Sickle cell	• Sickle cells/drepanocytes are **sickle**-shaped red cells found in sickle cell disease.
b	Target cell	• Target cell is a form of leptocyte in which there is **central** round stained area and a peripheral rim of hemoglobin. • Target cells are found in iron deficiency, thalassemia, chronic liver disease and after splenectomy.
c	Gaucher's cell	• Microscopy in Gaucher's disease shows large number of characteristically distended and enlarged macrophages called Gaucher cells. • These cells are found in spleen, liver, bone marrow and lymph nodes. • In case of neuronal involvement, they are found in Virchow-Robin space. • The cytoplasm of these cells is abundant, granular and fibrillary resembling **crumpled** tissue paper. • They have mostly a single nucleus but occasionally may have two or three nuclei.

Contd.

d	Hairy cell	• Hairy cells are abnormal mononuclear cells with hairy cytoplasmic **projections** which are seen in the bone marrow, peripheral smear and spleen, in a case of hairy cell leukaemia. • These cells are best recognised under phase contrast microscopy but may be visible in routine blood smears.

Coming back to the question:

- *Mononuclear cell with hairy cytoplasmic projections is known as hairy cell.*

10. Which of the following is a specific marker for alcoholic liver disease?

A. Serum bilirubin

B. Gamma-Glutamyl Transpeptidase

C. SGPT

D. SGOT

Key points about alcoholic liver disease/ALD:

- *There are 3 distinctive forms of ALD.*
- *Hepatocellular steatosis/Fatty change:*
  - o *Liver is enlarged, soft, yellow and greasy in consistency.*
  - o *Lipid droplets accumulate in hepatocytes.*
- *Alcoholic (or steato-) hepatitis:*
  - o *Hepatocytes swelling and necrosis.*
  - o *Mallory-Denk bodies: Eosinophilic material in hepatocytes, made up of intermediate filaments (keratins 8 and 18 in complex with ubiquitin).*
- *Alcoholic steatofibrosis:*
  - o *Due to activation of stellate cells and portal fibroblasts, with resultant fibrosis.*
  - o *Chicken wire fence pattern of scar.*
  - o *Laennec cirrhosis: End stage ALD.*

- *Clinical features:*
  - o *In ALD, serum AST levels are higher than serum ALT levels (2 : 1 ratio of higher).*
  - o *In other chronic liver diseases – Serum ALT tends to be higher than AST.*

Let's discuss the options:

Option	*Statement*	*Remarks*
a	Serum bilirubin	• Estimation of serum bilirubin is based on van den Bergh diazo reaction by spectrophotometric method. • Water-soluble conjugated bilirubin gives direct van den Bergh reaction with diazo reagent within one minute. • Whereas alcohol-soluble unconjugated bilirubin is determined by indirect van den Bergh reaction. • The serum of normal adults contains less than 1 mg/dl of total bilirubin, out of which less than 0.25 mg/dl is conjugated bilirubin. • Bilirubin level rises in diseases of hepatocytes, obstruction to biliary excretion into the duodenum, in hemolysis, and defects of hepatic uptake and conjugation of bilirubin pigment such as in Gilbert's disease.
b	Gamma-Glutamyl Transpeptidase (γ-GT)	• The primary source of γ-GT enzyme in serum is the liver. • Its serum level parallels serum alkaline phosphatase and is used to confirm that the elevated serum alkaline phosphatase is of hepatobiliary origin. • Besides its elevation in cholestasis and hepatocellular disease, the levels are high in patients with **alcohol** abuse even without liver disease.

Contd.

c	SGPT	• SGPT is also known as serum alanine transaminase/ALT/Glutamic pyruvic transaminase. • It is a cytosolic enzyme primarily present in the liver. • Serum SGPT, is of greater value in liver cell injury.
d	SGOT	• SGOT is also known as serum aspartate transaminase/AST/Glutamic oxaloacetic transaminase. • It is a mitochondrial enzyme released from heart, liver, skeletal muscle and kidney. • SGOT level may rise in acute necrosis or ischemia of other organs such as myocardium, besides liver cell injury.

Coming back to the question:

- *Gamma-Glutamyl Transpeptidase is a specific marker for alcoholic liver disease.*

11. Which of the following is the correct sequence of filling blood in vacutainer?

A. Grey – Red – Lavender – Blue
B. Red – Lavender – Grey – Blue
C. Blue – Lavender – Red – Grey
D. Blue – Red – Lavender – Grey

Key points about order of blood draw tubes:

- *Blood samples must be drawn by phlebotomists in a specific order to avoid cross-contamination of the sample by additives found in different collection tubes.*
- *Phlebotomy order of draw is the same for specimens collected by syringe, tube holder, or into tubes pre-evacuated at the time of collection.*
- *The correct order of draw is as follows:*

- o *Blood culture tube or bottle.*
- o *Sodium citrate tube (e.g.,* ***B****lue closure).*
- o *Serum tubes, including those with clot activator and gels (e.g.,* ***R****ed, red-speckled, gold closures).*
- o *Heparin tube with or without gel (e.g., dark* ***G****reen, light green, speckled green closures).*
- o *EDTA tube with or without gel separator (e.g.,* ***L****avender, pearl, pink closures).*
- o *Sodium fluoride/potassium oxalate glycolytic inhibitor (e.g.,* ***G****rey closure).*

Closure Color	Collection Tube	Mix by Inverting
	Blood Cultures	8 to 10 times
	Serum (glass tube)	—
	Citrate	3 to 4 times
	BD SST™ Gel Separator Tube	5 times
	BD SST Gel Separator Tube	"
	Serum (plastic tube)	"
	Heparin	8 to 10 times
	BD PST™ Gel Separator Tube With Heparin	"
	EDTA	8 to 10 times
	Fluoride (glucose tube)	8 to 10 times

Coming back to the question:

- *Correct order of filling blood in vacutainer is Blue – Red – Lavender – Grey.*

12. All of the following are true for BRCA-1 gene EXCEPT:

A. It causes ovarian carcinoma

B. It is a tumour suppressor gene

C. It is involved in repair of DNA in double strand breaks

D. It is mutated in Fanconi's anemia

Key points about BRCA genes:

- *BRCA 1 gene:*
    - o *Tumour-**suppressor** anti-oncogene.*
    - o *Located on chromosome 17q21, a DNA **repair** gene, is implicated in both breast and **ovarian** cancer in inherited cases.*
    - o *BRCA1 deletion is seen in about two-third of women with inherited breast cancer having family history but BRCA1 mutation is uncommon in sporadic cases.*
    - o *The protein product of BRCA gene is a cell cycle regulated protein and it can be detected by immunohistochemistry.*
    - o *Men who have mutated BRCA1 have increased risk of developing cancer of the prostate but not of male breast.*
- *BRCA 2 gene:*
    - o *Tumour-suppressor anti-oncogene.*
    - o *BRCA2 gene located on chromosome 13q12-13, another DNA repair gene, in its mutated form, has a similarly higher incidence of inherited cancer of the breast (one-third cases) and ovary in females and prostate in men.*

Coming back to the question:

- *Mutation of BRCA gene is not seen in Fanconi's anemia.*

13. Which type of amyloid is seen in renal dialysis?

A. AA B. AL

C. ATTR D. A-beta 2 microglobulin

Key points about amyloidosis:

- *Amyloid is a pathologic proteinaceous substance, which on Hematoxylin and Eosin (H and E) stain appears as amorphous, eosinophilic, hyaline and **extracellular** substance.*
- *First described by Rokitansky in 1842, the substance was subsequently named by Virchow as 'amyloid' under the mistaken belief that the material was **starch**-like (amylon = starch).*
- *This property was demonstrable grossly on the cut surface of an organ containing amyloid which stained brown with iodine and turned violet on addition of dilute sulphuric acid.*

- *Physical nature:*
  - o *X-ray crystallography: Shows characteristic cross* ***beta****-pleated sheet conformation.*
  - o *Electron microscopy: Amyloid appears as continuous, non-branching fibrils with a diameter of approximately 7.5 to 10 nm.*
- *Pathogenesis of amyloid:*
  - o *Results from abnormal folding of proteins, which gets deposited in extracellular tissues and disrupt normal function.*
- *Staining pattern:*
  - o ***Most*** *common staining technique: Congo red dye.*
  - o *Congo red under ordinary light, imparts pink or red colour to amyloid.*
  - o *Under polarized light Congo red-stained amyloid shows apple green birefringence.*
  - o *Other stains: Crystal violet and Thioflavin-T.*

Let's discuss the options:

Option	*Statement*	*Remarks*
a	AA	• Amyloid-associated protein. • Protein precursor is SAA (serum amyloid-associated) protein, synthesized in liver. • Seen in chronic inflammatory conditions (secondary amyloidosis).
b	AL	• Amyloid-light chain protein. • Protein precursor is monoclonal immuno-globulin light chain. • It is seen in multiple myeloma.
c	ATTR	• Transthyretin (TTR). • Binds and transports thyroxin and retinol. • Mutant form of TTR is deposited in familial amyloid polyneuropathies. • Normal TTR is deposited in heart of aged individuals (senile systemic amyloidosis).

Contd.

d	A-beta 2 micro-globulin	• It is found in patients on long-term **hemodialysis.**

Coming back to the question:

- *A-beta 2 microglobulin amyloid protein is found in renal dialysis patients.*

14. All of the following are true regarding amyloidosis EXCEPT:

A. Beta-pleated sheet on X-ray crystallography

B. Name amyloid is derived because of accumulation of starch

C. There is extracellular accumulation of protein

D. AL is seen in secondary type of amyloidosis

Key points about AL protein:

- *AL amyloid fibril protein is derived from immunoglobulin light chain, which may be complete light chain, or may include amino-terminal segment and part of C region of the immunoglobulin light chain.*
- *AL fibril protein is more frequently derived from the lambda light chain (twice more common) than kappa.*
- *AL type of fibril protein is produced by immunoglobulin secreting cells and is therefore seen in association with plasma cell dyscrasias and is induced in* **primary** *systemic amyloidosis.*

Coming back to the question:

- *AL is seen in primary type of amyloidosis (and not in secondary type of amyloidosis).*

15. Which of the following parameters are seen in iron deficiency anemia?

I. Low serum iron

II. Low serum ferritin

III. Low transferrin saturation

IV. Raised total iron binding capacity

Lead – Choose the best answer from the codes given below:

A. I and II
B. II and III
C. I, II and III
D. I, II, III and IV

Key points about iron deficiency anemia/IDA:

- ***Most*** *common nutritional disorder in the world.*
- *Clinical sign and symptoms are due to inadequate hemoglobin synthesis iron.*
- *Iron metabolism:*
  - o *Functional iron (80%) is found in hemoglobin, myoglobin, iron-containing enzymes such as catalase and cytochromes.*
  - o *Storage pool (20%) is hemosiderin and ferritin.*
  - o ***Major*** *site of iron storage is liver and mononuclear phagocytes.*
  - o *Iron is transported in plasma by transferrin (synthesized in liver).*
- *Cause of IDA:*
  - o *Dietary deficiency.*
  - o *Impaired iron absorption.*
  - o *Increased requirement.*
  - o *Chronic blood loss.*
- *1 mg of iron* ***must*** *be absorbed from the diet everyday.*
- *Absorption of inorganic iron:*
  - o *Increased by ascorbic acid, citric acid, amino acids, sugars in the diet.*
  - o *Inhibited by tannates (found in tea), carbonates, oxalates and phosphates.*

Let's discuss the options:

Option	***Statement***	***Remarks***
I	Low serum iron	• **True** statement. • In IDA, serum iron is **decreased** (< 30 μg/dL).

Contd.

II	Low serum ferritin	• **True** statement. • In IDA, serum ferritin is **low** (<12 μg/dL). • It is the first indication toward IDA.
III	Low transferrin saturation	• **True** statement. • Transferrin saturation (serum iron/TIBC × 100) is **less** than 15%.
IV	Raised total iron binding capacity	• **True** statement. • TIBC (total amount of iron in body that can bind to transferrin present in plasma) is **increased**.

Coming back to the question:

- *In IDA, serum iron, serum ferritin and transferrin saturation is low whereas TIBC is increased.*

16. Identify the ANA pattern shown below:

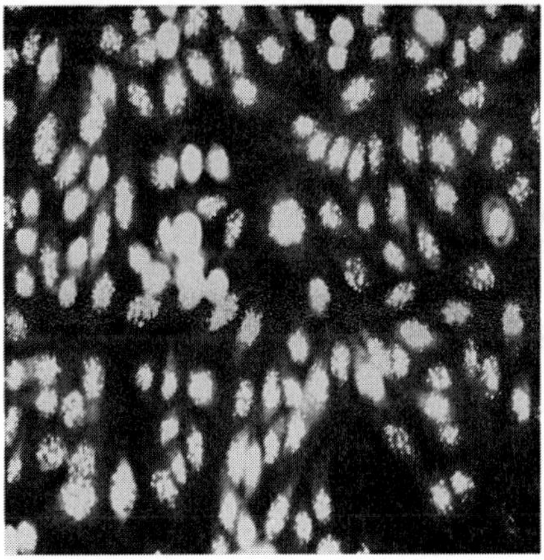

A. Centromeric
B. Homogenous
C. Speckled
D. Nucleolar

Key points about ANA/antinuclear antibodies:

- *These are the antibodies against common nuclear antigen that includes DNA as well as RNA.*
- *These are demonstrable in about 98% cases of SLE are used as screening test.*

Let's discuss the options:

Option	*Statement*	*Remarks*
a	Centromeric	• Centromeric pattern is seen in systemic sclerosis. • A centromere staining pattern means the ANA staining is present along the chromosomes.
b	Homogenous	• Homogenous/Diffuse nuclear staining pattern is seen in antibodies to chromatin, histones, dsDNA.
c	Speckled	• Speckled pattern antibodies to Sm antigen, RNP, SS-A and SS-B reactive antigens.
d	Nucleolar	• Nucleolar pattern represents antibodies to RNA. • Seen in patients with systemic sclerosis. • A nucleolar staining pattern means the ANA staining is present along the nucleolus.

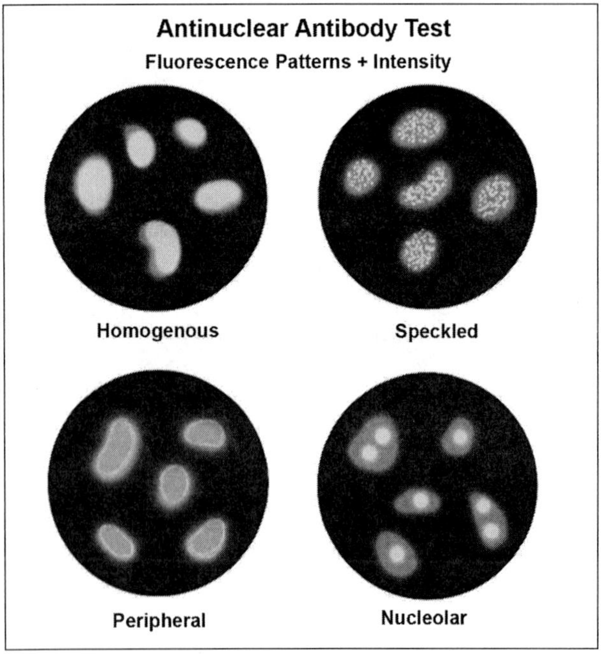

Coming back to the question:

- *ANA staining along the chromosomes suggest Centromeric pattern.*

17. A patient developed acute hepatitis B infection. This was followed by complete recovery. Sequence of serologic and viral markers is shown below. Green line represents which of the following marker?

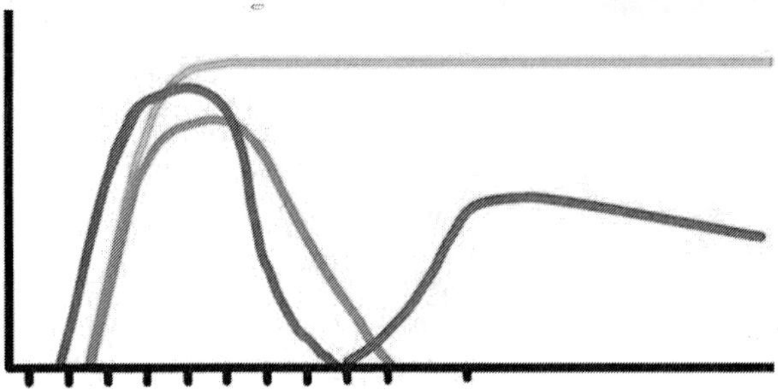

A. HBsAg
B. Anti-HBs
C. HBcAg
D. Anti-HBc

Key points about hepatitis B infection:

- *Hepatitis B virus:*
  - o *It belongs to Hepadnaviridae family.*
  - o *Spherical double layered 'Dane particle'.*
  - o *HBV genome contains envelope glycoproteins (HBsAg/ hepatitis B surface antigen), core protein (HBcAg/hepatitis B core antigen), pre-core and core region (HbeAg/hepatitis B 'envelope' antigen), polymerase (pol) that exhibits both DNA polymerase activity and reverse transcriptase activity and HBx protein (necessary for viral replication and it is implicated in hepatocellular carcinoma).*
- *Incubation period: 2-26 weeks (mean of 8 weeks).*
- *Mode of infection:*
  - o *Blood borne.*
  - o *During childbirth.*
  - o *Unprotected sex.*
  - o *Intravenous drug abuse.*
  - o *Blood transfusion.*

- *Natural course:*
  - o *HBsAg, HBeAg, HBV-DNA and DNA polymerase in the serum signify active viral replication.*
  - o *Persistence of HBeAg is an important indicator of continued viral replication.*

Let's discuss the options:

Option	*Statement*	*Remarks*
a	HBsAg	• HBsAg appears early in the blood and its detection is an indicator of active HBV infection. • It usually disappears in 3-6 months. • Its persistence for more than 6 months implies a carrier state. • Demonstrated by **blue** line in the graph given in the question.
b	Anti-HBs	• Specific antibody to HBsAg in serum called anti-HBs appears late. • Anti-HBs response may be both IgM and IgG type. • The prevalence rate of anti-HBs ranges from 10-15%. • In these individuals it persists for life providing protection against reinfection with HBV. • Demonstrated by **purple** line in the graph.
c	HBcAg	• HBcAg derived from core protein **cannot** be detected in blood.
d	Anti-HBc	• Antibody to HBcAg called anti-HBc can, however, be detected in the serum of acute hepatitis B patients during pre-icteric stage. • In the initial period, it is IgM class antibody which persists for 4-6 months and is followed later by IgG anti-HBc.

Contd.

		• Thus detection of high titre of IgM anti-HBc is indicative of recent acute HBV infection. • Elevated level of IgG anti-HBc suggests HBV infection in the remote past. • IgM anti-HBc is represented by **brown** line. • IgG anti-HBc is drawn in **green** color.

Coming back to the question:

- ***Blue*** *line in the diagram represents* ***HBsAg.***
- ***Green*** *line in the diagram represents* ***IgG anti-HBc.***
- ***Brown*** *line in the diagram represents* ***IgM anti-HBc.***
- ***Purple*** *line in the diagram represents* ***anti-HBs.***

MICROBIOLOGY

1. CD40 gene mutation is seen in:

A. Common Variable Immunodeficiency
B. Hyper-IgM syndrome
C. Bruton disease
D. Transient hypogammaglobulinemia of infancy

Let's discuss the options:

Option	*Statement*	*Remarks*
a	Common Variable Immunodeficiency	• This is a heterogeneous group of both sporadic and inherited forms of the disease characterized by hypogammaglobulinemia, increased susceptibility to infection, auto-immune disorders (hemolytic anemia, pernicious anemia), as well as lymphoid tumours. • Both sexes are affected equally. • Onset of symptoms is much later, in the second or third decade. • It is a B-cell development defect. • B-cells may be present in circulation in normal numbers, but they appear defective in their ability to differentiate into plasma cells and secrete immunoglobulins. • The diagnosis is usually one of **exclusion** (after other cause of immunodeficiency are ruled out). • The basis of the immunoglobulin deficiency is variable (hence the name).

Contd.

		• The defect in the antibody production has been variably attributed to intrinsic B-cell defects, deficient T-cell help, or excessive T-cell suppressor activity.
b	Hyper-IgM syndrome	• It is a X-linked disorder; results due to a defect in isotype class switchover of B-cells. • Class switchover is a phenomenon by which the same B-cell, instead of producing IgM, starts producing other classes of antibodies. • Class switchover depends upon two signals generated by helper T-cells which influence the B-cells: (1) T_H cell induced cytokine; (2) signal generated due to direct contact through the interaction of CD40 molecules on B-cells with CD40 ligand (CD40L) on T_H cells. • In hyper-IgM syndrome, there occur **mutations** in either CD40L or CD40 genes; prevent the T- and B-cell interaction; thus blocking the class switchover. • A block in class switchover results in lack of synthesis of other classes of antibodies such as IgG, IgA, and IgE with a normal or supernormal levels of IgM. • Because CD40L signals are involved in macrophage activation and thus producing delayed hypersensitivity response, hence patients with defect in CD40L are **more** susceptible to *Pneumocytis jirovecii* infection.

Contd.

c	Bruton disease	• It is one of the **more** common forms of primary immunodeficiency. • It is characterized by failure of pre-B-cells to differentiate into immature B-cells in the bone marrow – due to the absence of an enzyme called Bruton's tyrosine kinase which is involved in transformation of pre-B-cell into immature B-cell. • As a result, there occur total absence of B-cells and plasma cells in the circulation, with depressed serum levels of all classes of immunoglobulins. • However, Pre-B-cells are found in normal numbers in bone marrow and the T-cell-mediated responses are also normal. • The B-cell maturation stops at pre-B-cell stage; after the synthesis of heavy-chain without forming the light chains. • Hence the cytoplasm of pre-B-cell may have incomplete immunoglobulins. • Secondary infections are seen after 6 months of age, when maternal antibodies are depleted.
d	Transient hypogammaglobulinemia of infancy	• This occurs due to an abnormal delay in the initiation of synthesis of IgG (or some time IgA or IgM). • IgG synthesis usually starts by 2 months of age. But in some infants, it is delayed leading to defect in opsonisation or complement activation resulting in recurrent otitis media and respiratory infections.

Contd.

		• However, spontaneous recovery occurs usually by 18-24 months of age. • Interestingly, these infant show a **normal** antibody response against vaccines.

Coming back to the question:

- *CD40 gene mutation is seen in Hyper-IgM syndrome.*

2. Match the following:

Diseases	*Incubation period*
1. Hepatitis A virus	**A. 14-21 days**
2. Chickenpox	**B. 10 days**
3. Covid-19	**C. 15-45 days**
4. Syphilis	**D. 9-90 days**

Lead – Choose the best answer from the codes given below:

A. 1-B, 2-A, 3-D, 4-C
B. 1-C, 2-B, 3-A, 4-D
C. 1-A, 2-B, 3-C, 4-D
D. 1-C, 2-A, 3-B, 4-D

Let's discuss the options:

Option	*Statement*	*Remarks*
1	Hepatitis A virus	• HAV belongs to the family Picornaviridae. • It was originally designated as 'enterovirus 72', but based on the nucleotide and amino acid sequences, it was later assigned to a new genus, Hepatovirus under Picornaviridae family. • HAV is transmitted principally by feco-oral route. • Children and adolescents (5-14 years) are most commonly affected, majority remains subclinical (80-95%), but excrete virus in feces for longer time. • Adults are more icteric (75-90%) than children with **higher** mortality rate.

Contd.

		• Outbreaks are **common** in summer camps, day care centers, families and institutions, neonatal ICUs, and among military troops. • Incubation period is about **5-45** days (mean 30 days). • Onset is relatively abrupt (subacute).
2	Chickenpox	• Chickenpox is caused by VZV. • Varicella-zoster virus (VZV) produces vesicular eruptions (rashes) on the skin and mucous membranes in the form of two clinical entities: (1) Chickenpox, which is characterized by generalized diffuse bilateral vesicular rashes which occur following primary infection, usually affecting children. (2) Zoster/ shingles occurs following reactivation of latent VZV, present in the trigeminal ganglia that occurs mainly in adult life. Vesicular rashes are unilateral and segmental (confined to the skin innervated by a single sensory ganglion). • Incubation period of chickenpox is about **10-21** days (2-3 weeks). • Rashes of chickenpox are vesicular, centripetal in distribution (start on the face and trunk, spread rapidly to involve flexor surfaces), bilateral and diffuse in distribution and appears in multiple crops (lesions in various stages of evolution, such as maculopapules, vesicles, and scabs can be found in one area at the same time).
3	Covid-19	• Covid-19 is caused by a strain of coronavirus, SARS-CoV-2 (Severe Acute Respiratory Syndrome). • Coronaviruses are enveloped; carrying petal or club-shaped or crown-like peplomer spikes giving appearance of solar corona.

Contd.

		• They are large (120-160 nm) spherical viruses having a helical symmetry. • They possess linear, positive-sense ssRNA of 26-32 kbp size, largest among the non-segmented RNA viruses. • Incubation period of Covid-19 is **2-14** days.
4	Syphilis	• Syphilis is caused by Treponema pallidum. • The name pallidum refers to pale-staining property. • Treponemes are extremely thin and delicate with tapering ends. • They are flexible, spirally coiled around the long axis; possess 6-14 spirals spaced at intervals of 1 μm with amplitude of 1-1.5 μm. • They are actively motile exhibiting flexion extension, translatory, and cork-screw motility. They have a typical tendency to bend at right angle at the midpoint. • Treponemes **cannot** be visualized by light microscope but can be seen under dark ground or phase contrast microscope. • They do **not** take up ordinary stain but can be stained by fluorescence staining and the silver impregnation methods (which increase the thickness of the bacilli). • Incubation period of syphilis is variable (**9-90 days**) and is inversely proportional to the number of organisms inoculated. The median incubation period in humans is about 21 days which corresponds to an average inoculum of 500-1000 infectious organisms.

Coming back to the question:

Diseases	*Incubation period*
1. Hepatitis A virus	*C. 15-45 days*
2. Chickenpox	*A. 14-21 days*
3. Covid-19	*B. 10 days*
4. Syphilis	*D. 9-90 days*

3. Which of the protozoan pathogen is found in Kupffer cells of liver?

A. Giardia lamblia
B. Leishmania
C. Babesia microtii
D. Plasmodium vivax

Let's discuss the options:

Option	*Statement*	*Remarks*
a	Giardia lamblia	• Giardia is the **only** protozoan parasite found in the lumen of the human **small intestine** (duodenum and jejunum). • Trophozoites are pear-shaped, bilaterally symmetrical with 2 nuclei, 4 pairs of flagella, and a ventral concave sucking disc. • Trophozoites exhibit motility resembling a 'falling leaf'. • Ellipsoid cysts contain 4 nuclei with remnants of flagella.
b	Leishmania	• Visceral leishmaniasis (Kala azar) is caused by L. donovani and L. infantum. • Vector of Kala azar is female sandfly (Phlebotomus species). • **Definitive host:** Man, dog and other animals. • **Infective form:** Promastigote form present in midgut of female sand-fly. • Kala azar is reticuloendotheliosis resulting from the invasion of reticulo-endothelial system by L. donovani.

Contd.

		• Amastigote forms (LD body) is found in macrophages and monocytes in human. • In liver, the **Kupffer** cells and vascular endothelial cells are heavily parasitized, but hepatocytes are not affected. • Liver function is, therefore **not** seriously affected, although prothrombin production is commonly decreased. • The sinusoidal capillaries of liver are dilated and engorged. • Some degree of fatty degeneration is seen. The cut surface may show a 'nutmeg' appearance. • The liver is enlarged.
c	Babesia microtii	• Babesia are intra-erythrocytic sporozoan parasites that morphologically resemble plasmodium and cause tick-borne malaria like illness in domestic and wild animals. • It causes opportunistic infection in humans. • **Definitive host:** Ixodid ticks. • **Intermediate host:** Man or other mammals. • **Infective form:** Sporozoites (for humans). • Sporozoites present in the salivary glands of salivary glands of tick are introduced in man or other animals (intermediate host). • Sporozoites change to trophozoites in the circulation, which then invade the **RBCs** and multiple asexually by binary fission or schizogony to form 4 or more trophozoites. • Newly formed trophozoites are released by rupturing erythrocytes and invade new erythrocytes.

Contd.

d	Plasmodium vivax	• Malarial parasites pass its life cycle in 2 hosts: o **Definitive host:** Female anopheles' mosquito. o **Intermediate host:** Man. • The life cycle of malarial parasite comprises 2 stages: An asexual phase occurring in humans, which act as the intermediate host and a sexual phase occurring in mosquito, which serves as a definitive host for the parasite. • In asexual stage, the malarial parasite multiplies by division or splitting, a process designated to as Schizogony. • In humans, schizogony occurs in two locations – in the **RBC**/red blood cell (erythrocytic schizogony) and in the liver cells (exoerythrocytic schizogony/tissue phase). • Because schizogony in the liver is an essential step before the parasites can invade erythrocytes, it is called pre-erythrocytic schizogony. • Within an hour of being injected into the body by the mosquito, the sporozoites reach the liver and enter the **hepatocytes** to initiate the stage of pre-erythrocytic schizogony/merogony.

Coming back to the question:

- *Kupffer cells (liver macrophages) are parasitized by Leishmania donovani.*

4. A patient on ventilator developed pneumonia. Critical care physician isolates an organism which is gram-negative and susceptible to co-trimoxazole and ticarcillin/clavulanic acid but resistant to many other antibiotics. The organism in consideration is:

A. Acinetobacter
B. Stenotrophomonas maltophilia
C. Burkholderia cepacia
D. Pseudomonas aeruginosa

Let's discuss the options:

Option	*Statement*	*Remarks*
a	Acinetobacter	• Acinetobacter are saprophytic bacilli, present in the environment (soil, water and phytosphere). • However, during the last two decades, it has gained increasing attention as nosocomial pathogen. • Unhygienic practices in hospitals (contaminated hands of staff) and warm hospital environment (summers) promote colonization. • Patients with underlying diseases or immunosuppression are predisposed to invasion and pathogenesis. • Its ability to develop drug resistance rapidly to almost all available antibiotics makes it dangerous in hospital settings. • *Acinetobacter baumanii* causes widespread hospital infections such as ventilator associated pneumonia, central line associated blood stream infection, post-neurosurgical meningitis, catheter associated UTI etc. • Acinetobacter is notorious to develop resistance to multiple drugs including beta-lactams, aminoglycosides and quinolones.

Contd.

		• Beta-lactam resistance can be attributed to production of beta-lactamases such as metallo-beta-lactamases (MBL), AmpC-beta-lactamases and OXA-type beta-lactamases. • Common antibiotics indicated in management are **fluoroquinolones**, carbapenems, amikacin, tigecycline and colistin.
b	Stenotrophomonas maltophilia	• S. maltophilia is a saprophyte found in the rhizosphere (soil surrounding the plant roots). • **Pathogenesis:** It is mediated by the host's inflammatory response to components of the organism such as LPS and flagellin. • **Drug resistance:** It is resistant to most of the antibiotics. Beta-lactam resistance is efflux pump mediated. • The recommended antibiotics are **co-trimoxazole**, ticarcillin/clavulanate and levofloxacin. • **Clinical manifestations:** S. maltophilia can cause various hospital infections such as pneumonia in ventilated patients, blood stream infections and ecthyma gangrenosum in neutropenic patients.
c	Burkholderia cepacia	• *B. cepacia* is currently the most commonly encountered Burkholderia species. • It is an environmental organism that inhabits moist environments, detergents and IV fluids. • **Cepacia syndrome:** It is characterized by a rapidly fatal respiratory infection and septicaemia in patients with cystic fibrosis.

Contd.

		• **Nosocomial pathogen:** It is resistant to multiple antibiotics, hence has been emerging as an important nosocomial pathogen in ICUs causing pneumonia, wound infections etc. • B. cepacia is intrinsically resistant to many antibiotics. Therefore, treatment must be based on the sensitivity report. • **Co-trimoxazole**, meropenem and doxycycline are the most effective agents.
d	Pseudomonas aeruginosa	• Pseudomonas is an oxidase positive, pigment producing, non-fermenting gram-negative bacilli. • It is a major pathogen among the hospitalized patients and in patients with cystic fibrosis. • *Pseudomonas aeruginosa* is notorious to cause infections at almost all sites, most common being lungs, skin and soft tissues. • Most of the infections are encountered in hospitalized patients who get colonized with the organisms either from heavily contaminated hospital environment or from the hospital staff (through contaminated hands). • Colonized patients develop disease in the presence of underlying risk factors such as burn wounds, patients with immunosuppression and post-surgeries. • **VAP** (ventilator associated pneumonia): It develops among the patients on ventilator in intensive care units.

Contd.

		• Chronic respiratory tract infections occur in patients with underlying conditions such as cystic fibrosis (in Caucasian populations), bronchiectasis or chronic panbronchiolitis (in Japan). • Pseudomonas species are inherently resistant to most of the antibiotics. • Only **limited** antimicrobial agents have antipseudomonal action, such as: o **Penicillin:** Piperacillin, mezlocillin, ticarcillin. o **Cephalosporin: Ceftazidime**, cefoperazone and cefepime. o **Carbapenem:** Imipenem, meropenem. o **Monobactam:** Aztreonam. o **Aminoglycosides:** Tobramycin, gentamicin, amikacin. o **Quinolones:** Ciprofloxacin, levofloxacin.

5. A young patient presented with subacute onset of cough with thick, purulent sputum. The organism recovered from sputum was gram-positive, aerobic and acid fast. The microscopic image is shown below. Most likely organism is:

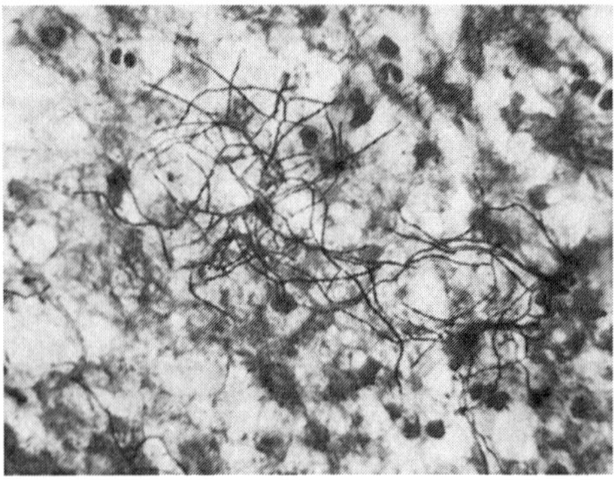

A. Actinomyces B. Nocardia
C. Pneumococcus D. Listeria

Clinical presentation is indicative of lobar pneumonia.

Let's discuss the options:

Option	*Statement*	*Remarks*
a	Actinomyces	• Actinomyces are soil saprophytes and commensals of oral cavity. • The name refers to ray-like appearance of the organism in the granules (*Actinomyces*, meaning ray fungus). • *A. israelii* is the **most** common species infecting man. • In humans, they cause actinomycosis. • Actinomycosis is a chronic suppurative and granulomatous infection characterized by multiple abscesses with formation of sinuses, discharge containing granules and on later stage; fibrosis and tissue destruction. • Cervical actinomycosis is the **most** common form, usually presents as a painless, slow-growing, hard mass with cutaneous fistulas, a condition commonly known as lumpy jaw. • Gram staining (Brown-Brenn modification) shows a central mass of gram-positive filamentous bacilli, radiating peripherally with hyaline, club-shaped ends.
b	Nocardia	• Nocardia species (named after Edmond Nocard, 1898) are gram-positive branching filamentous bacilli similar to Actinomyces; however, they differ from the later by being aerobic and acid-fast. • Lobar pneumonia is the **most** common form of pulmonary nocardiosis.

Contd.

		• In half of the cases of pulmonary nocardiosis, dissemination occurs via blood. • Gram staining (Brown-Brenn modification) shows gram-positive branching and filamentous bacilli. • Modified acid-fast staining using 1% sulphuric acid as decolorizer (Kinyoun method) demonstrates nocardia as partially **acid-fast**. They appear as branching and filamentous red colored acid-fast bacilli.
c	Pneumococcus	• *Streptococcus pneumoniae* (commonly referred to as pneumococcus) is the **leading** cause of lobar pneumonia, otitis media in children and meningitis in all ages. • Direct microscopy of smears made from sputum, pus or CSF shows numerous pus cells and lanceolate or flame shaped gram-positive cocci in pairs, surrounded by a clear halo (due to capsule).
d	Listeria	• *Listeria monocytogenes* is a food-borne pathogen that causes serious infections, particularly in neonates, pregnant women and elderly people. • **Gram stain:** Gram-positive short coccobacilli, often confused with diphtheroids.

Coming back to the question:

- *Gram-positive, aerobic and acid fast organism causing lobar pneumonia is Nocardia.*

6. A patient presented with multiple liver abscesses in the upper right lobe of the liver, with irregular margins. There is a past history of bloody dysentery. Most likely diagnosis:

A. Hydatid cyst B. Pyogenic liver abscess
C. Typhoid D. Amoebiasis

Let's discuss the options:

Option	*Statement*	*Remarks*
a	Hydatid cyst	• **Most** of the times infection is asymptomatic and accidentally discovered. • Clinical disease develops only when the hydatid cyst has grown big enough to cause obstructive symptoms. • In about half the cases, the primary hydatid cyst occurs in liver (63%), mostly in the right lobe. • Hepatomegaly, pain and obstructive jaundice are the usual manifestations.
b	Pyogenic liver abscess	• Pyogenic liver abscess is characterized by pain in the right upper quadrant, fever, tender hepatomegaly and sometimes jaundice. • They occur as single or multiple abscesses, 1 cm or more in diameter, in an enlarged liver. • A single abscess generally has a thick fibrous capsule. • The abscesses are particularly **common** in right lobe of the liver.
c	Typhoid	• Incubation period of enteric fever is 10-14 days. • Enteric fever is a misnomer as the manifestations are more extra-intestinal than intestinal. • Fever (step ladder pattern type or remittent fever). • Rashes (rose spots). • Abdominal pain, nausea, vomiting and anorexia. • Hepatosplenomegaly, epistaxis and relative bradycardia. • Gastrointestinal bleeding and intestinal perforation can occur **mostly** in the third and fourth week of illness.

Contd.

d	Amoebiasis	• The typical manifestation of intestinal amoebiasis is amoebic **dysentery**. • It is usually insidious in onset and the abdominal tenderness is less and localized (as compared to bacillary dysentery). • The stools are large, foul-smelling and brownish black, often with blood-streaked mucus intermingled with feces. • The RBCs in stools are clumped and reddish brown in color. Charcot-Leyden crystals are often present. • Hepatic involvement is the **most** common extra-intestinal complications of amoebiasis. • In about 5-10% of persons with intestinal amoebiasis, liver abscesses may ensue. The center of the abscess contains thick chocolate brown pus (anchovy sauce pus), which is liquefied necrotic liver tissue. • **Liver abscesses** may be multiple or more often solitary, usually located in the upper right lobe of the liver.

Coming back to the question:

- *Liver abscess with dysentery suggest the diagnosis of amoebiasis.*

7. A diabetic patient having an immunocompromised state presented with white, adherent, painless patches in mouth. Gram staining image is shown below. Most likely organism:

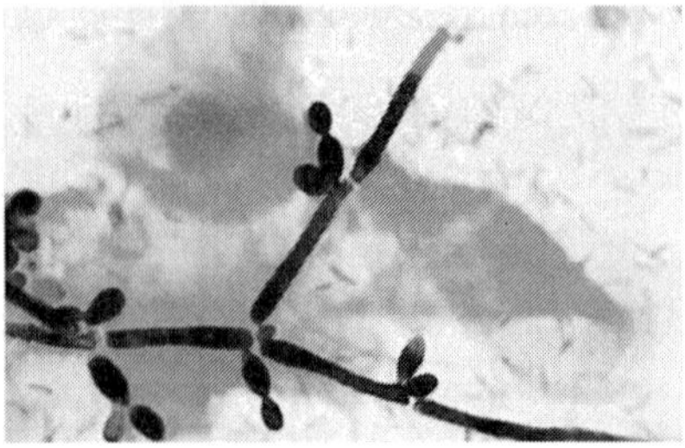

A. Cryptococcus B. Candida
C. Pneumocystis D. Aspergillus

Let's discuss the options:

Option	*Statement*	*Remarks*
a	Cryptococcus	• Cryptococcus is a capsulated yeast which is capable of producing potentially fatal meningitis in HIV infected people. • In people with low immunity, pulmonary infection occurs followed by dissemination through blood. • Pulmonary cryptococcosis is the **first** and the **most** common presentation. • **Cryptococcal meningitis:** It presents as chronic meningitis, with headache, fever, sensory and memory loss, cranial nerve paresis and loss of vision (due to optic nerve involvement). • Gram staining may show gram-positive round budding yeast cells.
b	Candida	• Predisposing factors that are associated with increased risk of infection with *Candida* include extremes of age, patients on steroid/**immunosuppressive** drugs, post-transplantation, malignancy, HIV infected people, **diabetic** patients etc. • Oropharyngeal candidiasis (**oral thrush**) presents as white, adherent, painless patches in mouth. • **Direct microscopy:** Gram staining reveals gram-positive **oval** budding yeast cells with pseudo-hyphae.
c	Pneumocystis	• Pneumocystis pneumonia (PcP) has been increasingly reported after the discovery of HIV/AIDS.

Contd.

		• Recently the taxonomy of *Pneumocystis* has been changed (2002). • One thought to be a protozoan, now it is classified under fungus based on nucleic acid sequence studies. • Taxonomists renamed the human species of *Pneumocystis* as *Pneumocystis jirovecii.* • The previously used species name *Pneumocystis* carinii has been assigned to describe the rate species of *Pneumocystis.* • Histopathological examination of lung tissue or fluid obtained by bronchoscopy, bronchial lavage, or open lung biopsy reveals cysts. • Gomori's methenamine silver (GMS) staining is the method of **choice** to demonstrate the cysts of *Pneumocystis jirovecii.* • The cysts resemble black colored crushed ping-pong balls, against the green background.
d	Aspergillus	• Risk factors for invasive aspergillosis are: Glucocorticoid use (most important risk factor), profound neutropenia, neutrophil dysfunction etc. • Aspergillosis refers to the invasive and allergic diseases caused by a hyaline mold named Aspergillus. • Pulmonary aspergillosis is the **most** common form of aspergillosis. • **Direct examination:** 10% KOH mount or histological staining of specimens reveals characteristic narrow septate hyaline hyphae with acute angle branching.

Coming back to the question:

- *In a diabetic, immunocompromised patient, white, adherent, painless patches in mouth, suggest the diagnosis of oropharyngeal candidiasis (oral thrush).*

8. Cat faeces is known to transmit toxoplasmosis. What is the infective form of toxoplasmosis, present in cat faeces?

A. Oocyst

B. Tachyzoite

C. Bradyzoite

D. Sporozoite

Key points about morphology of Toxoplasma gondii:

- *T. gondii occurs in 3 forms:*
  - o *Trophozoite.*
  - o *Tissue cyst.*
  - o *Oocyst.*
- *The trophozoite and tissue cyst represents stages in asexual multiplication (schizogony).*
- *Oocyst is formed by sexual reproduction (gametogony or sporogony).*
- *All 3 forms occur in domestic cats and other felines, which are the definitive hosts and support both schizogony and gametogony.*
- *Only the asexual forms, trophozoites and tissue cysts present in other animals, including humans and birds, which are the intermediate hosts.*

Let's discuss the options:

Option	***Statement***	***Remarks***
a, d	Oocyst, Sporozoites	• Oocyst develop **only** in definitive hosts – in the intestine of cats and other felines but not in humans. • They are formed by sexual reproduction (gametogony). • Cats shed millions of oocyts per day in **feces** for about 2 weeks during the primary infection. • The freshly passes oocyst is not infectious.

Contd.

		• They undergo sporulation in the soil with formation of 2 sporocysts, each containing 4 sporozoites. • The sporulated oocyst is **infective**. • When the infective oocyst is ingested, it releases sporozoites in the intestine, which initiates infection.
b	Tachyzoite	• Trophozoites/Tachyzoites is crescent shaped, with one end pointed and the other end rounded. • The nucleus is ovoid and is situated at the blunt end of the parasite. • The actively multiplying trophozoite is seen intracellularly in various **tissues** during early acute phase of infection. • The rapidly proliferating trophozoites in acute infection are called tachyzoites.
c	Bradyzoite	• **Tissue** cysts are the resting form of the parasite. • They are found during chronic stage of the infection and can be found in the brain (**most** common site), skeletal muscles and various other organs. • With periodic acid Schiff/PAS stain, the cyst walls stains weakly, and the parasites inside are stained deeply. • The slowly multiplying parasites within the cyst are called bradyzoites.

Coming back to the question:

- *Infective form of Toxoplasma gondii, present in cat feces is oocyst (sporulated).*

9. Identify the bacteria shown in the image below:

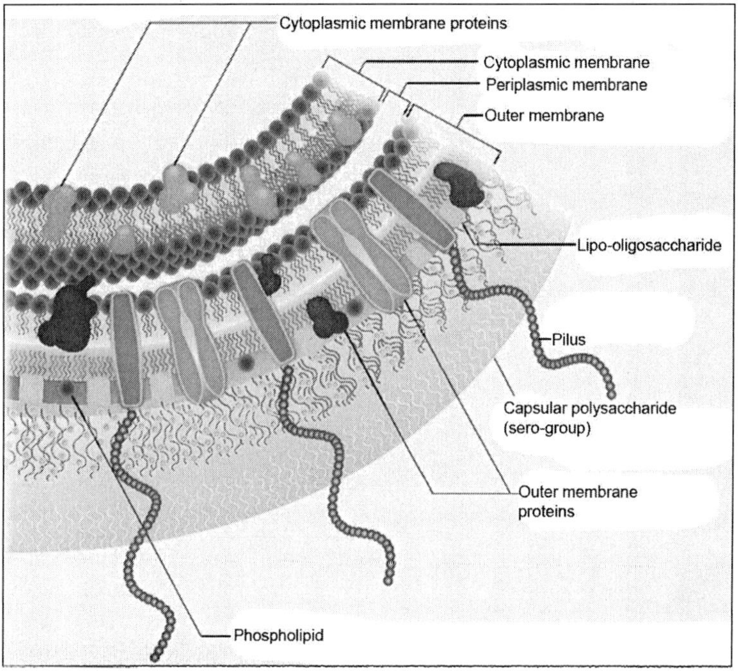

A. Staphylococcus aureus
B. Pseudomonas aeruginosa
C. Neisseria meningitidis
D. Escherichia coli

Let's discuss the options:

Option	*Statement*	*Remarks*
a	Staphylococcus aureus	• Staphylococcus aureus is catalase positive, coagulase positive, facultative anaerobe, non-motile, non-sporing and **occasionally** capsulated. • They are spherical cocci, about 1 μm in diameter, arranged in grape-like clusters. This arrangement is due to cell-division in *S. aureus* occurs in multiple planes with daughter cells remaining close to each other.

Contd.

		• Like most gram-positive bacteria, the cell wall of Staphylococcus consists of a thick peptidoglycan layer and teichoic acid. • *S. aureus* has additional factors in the cell wall, such as protein A and clumping factor. • Some strains of *S. aureus* have polysaccharide microcapsule, which inhibits phagocytosis by neutrophils.
b	Pseudomonas aeruginosa	• Pseudomonas is an oxidase positive, pigment producing, non-fermenting, gram-negative bacilli. • Many strains of Pseudomonas possess polysaccharide capsule, which prevents the bacteria from phagocytosis.
c	Neisseria meningitidis	• Meningococci are capsulated gram-negative diplococci with adjacent sides flattened (lens or half-moon shaped), present inside the polymorphs, often extracellular also. • **Capsular polysaccharide** is the **principal** virulence factor of meningococci; protects the bacteria from complement-mediated phagocytosis. • **Outer membrane proteins:** They are the porin proteins present beneath the capsule, embedded in the outer membrane. • There are of two types – PorA and PorB; both show antigenic variability and are responsible for serotyping (PorB) and subserotyping (PorA) of meningococci.

Contd.

d	Escherichia coli	• Gram-negative bacilli. • Aerobes and facultative anaerobes. • Non-fastidious, can grow in ordinary media like nutrient agar. • Ferment glucose to produce acid with or without gas. • Reduce nitrate to nitrite. • Produce catalase. • Do not produce oxidase. • Motile with peritrichous flagella.

Key points about:

- *Capsular polysaccharide and outer membrane proteins (Porin) are present in meningococci.*

10. A patient developed fever and pulmonary infiltrates after a heart transplant surgery. KOH smear of the sputum revealed oval budding yeast cells with pseudo-hyphae. Most likely diagnosis:

A. Histoplasmosis
B. Aspergillosis
C. Candidiasis
D. Cryptococcosis

Key points about hyphae and pseudo-hyphae:

- *Hyphae:*
  - o *Molds grow as long branching filaments of 2-10 μm wide called hyphae.*
  - o *Hyphae are either septate (i.e., form transverse walls) or non-septate (there are no transverse walls and they are multinucleated, i.e., coenocytic).*
  - o *Hyphae grow continuously and form a branching tangled mass of growth called mycelium.*
- *Pseudo-hyphae:*
  - o *In some yeast-like fungi (e.g., Candida), the bud remains attached to the mother cell, elongates and undergoes repeated budding to form chains of elongated cells known as pseudo-hyphae.*

- o *They can be differentiated from true hyphae as they have constriction at the septa and bear septa even at branching points.*

Let's discuss the options:

Option	***Statement***	***Remarks***
a	Histoplasmosis	• Classical histoplasmosis ranges from asymptomatic infection (in immuno-competent people) to life-threatening illness seen in people with low CMI. • Pulmonary histoplasmosis is the **most** common form of histoplasmosis. • Acute form presents with mild flu like illness, pulmonary infiltrates in chest X-ray with hilar or mediastinal lymphadenopathy. • **Direct microscopy:** Histopathological staining (such as PAS, Giemsa or GMS stain) of the specimens reveals tiny oval yeast cells (2-4 μm size) with narrow based budding within the macrophages with an underlying granulomatous response.
b	Aspergillosis	• **Direct examination:** 10% KOH mount or histological staining of specimens reveals characteristic narrow septate hyaline **hyphae** with acute angle branching.
c	Candidiasis	• Predisposing factors that are associated with increased risk of infection with *Candida* include extremes of age, patients on steroid/ immunosuppressive drugs, **post-transplantation**, malignancy, HIV infected people, diabetic patients etc. • Invasive candidiasis results from hematogenous or local spread of the fungi. Pulmonary candidiasis is one of the forms of invasive candidiasis.

Contd.

		• **Direct microscopy:** Gram staining reveals gram-positive **oval budding yeast** cells with **pseudo-hyphae**.
d	Cryptococcosis	• Cryptococcus is a capsulated yeast which is capable of producing potentially fatal meningitis in HIV infected people. • In people with low immunity, pulmonary infection occurs followed by dissemination through blood. • Gram staining may show gram-positive round budding yeast cells.

Coming back to the question:

- *Infection, after transplantation surgery and KOH smear demonstrating oval budding yeast cell with pseudo-hyphae suggest the diagnosis of candidiasis.*

11. A person who had splenectomy 5 years back, has a dog-bite. Tiny puncture wound and erythema was noted at the site of bite. The dog and the person were fully immunized. Next step in management:

A. Observation
B. Amoxyclav
C. Metronidazole
D. Ciprofloxacin

Clinical presentation is indicative of Pasteurella infection.

Key points about Pasteurella:

- *Pasteurella species are primarily harboured in respiratory tract of many animals and some time cause fatal diseases including hemorrhagic septicemia in animals.*
- *Pasteurella multocida is probably the most common organism in human wounds inflicted by the bites of cats and **dogs**.*
- *Pasteurella aviseptica is the chicken cholera bacillus, used by Louis Pasteur for the development of first attenuated bacterial vaccine hence the name Pasteurella was coined.*

- *Following animal* ***bite*** *(most common mode of transmission), the affected area becomes* ***red****, swollen and painful with variable regional lymphadenopathy and low grade fever.*
- *Direct microscopy of wound swabs shows non-motile gram-negative coccobacilli with a bipolar staining.*
- ***Culture:*** *They are aerobes or facultative anaerobes that grow readily on ordinary media like nutrient agar at 37° C.*
- *Most Pasteurella isolated are susceptible to oral antimicrobials such as amoxicillin, amoxicillin/clavulanic acid, tetracyclines etc.*

Coming back to the question:

- *Treatment of choice for Pasteurella infection is Amoxyclav.*

12. A child developed disseminated abscesses and granulomas in multiple organs. Morphology of the bacteria isolated is shown below in the image. Which of the following option is true for the bacteria isolated?

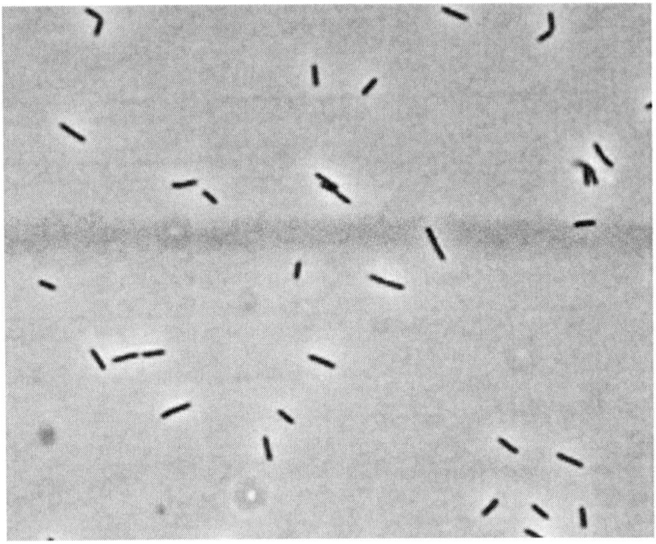

A. Gram-positive coccobacilli; motile at 25 degrees C; non-motile at 37 degrees C

B. Gram-positive coccobacilli; non-motile at 25 degrees C; motile at 37 degrees C

C. Gram-negative coccobacilli; motile at 25 degrees C; non-motile at 37 degrees C

D. Gram-negative coccobacilli; non-motile at 25 degrees C; motile at 37 degrees C

Clinical presentation is indicative of granulomatosis infantiseptica.

Key points about early onset neonatal listeriosis:

- *Caused by listeria monocytogenes:*
  - o *It is gram-positive short coccobacilli, often confused with diphtheroids.*
  - o *It shows tumbling type of motility at 25⁰ C but non-motile at 37⁰ C (**differential** motility), which is due to temperature dependent flagella expression.*
- *Occurs <5 days of age (mean age 1.5 days).*
- *Acquired from maternal genital flora.*
- *Associated with obstetrical complications like premature delivery and low birth weight.*
- ***Most** common form is neonatal sepsis.*
- *Granulomatosis infantiseptica:*
  - o *Occurs **rarely.***
  - o *Characterized by military microabscesses and granulomas, mostly in skin, liver and spleen.*
- *Mortality rate is >30%.*
- *Does **not** cause nosocomial break.*

Coming back to the question:

- *Granulomatosis infantiseptica is caused by listeria monocytogenes, a gram-positive coccobacilli, which is motile at 25⁰ C and non-motile at 37⁰ C.*

13. A 40 years old patient from south India, a cattle breeder, presented with a mass protruding from the nose. Clinical and histopathological image is shown below. Most likely pathogen:

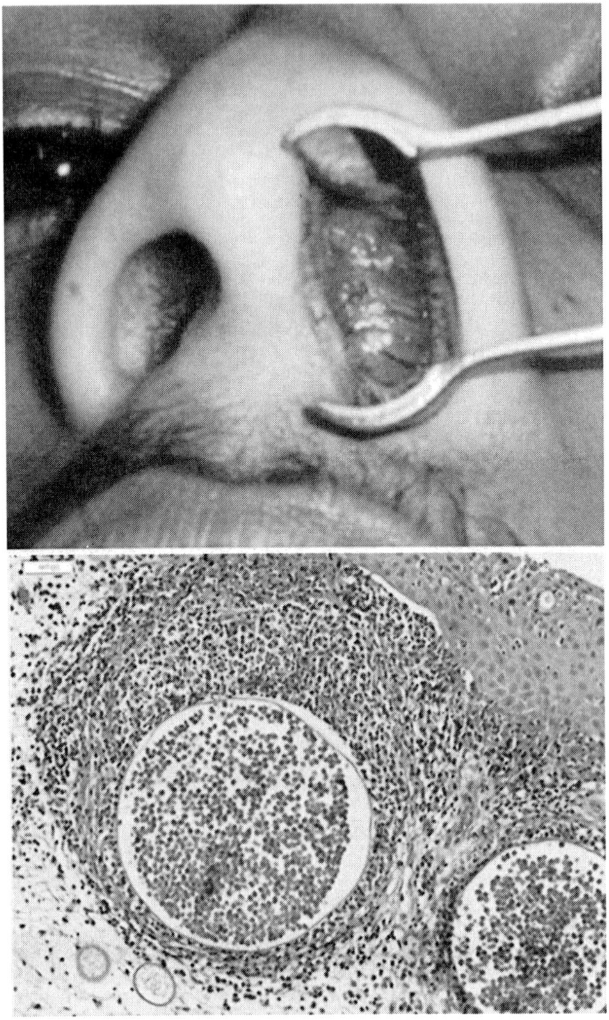

A. Klebsiella rhinoscleromatis

B. Mycobacterium tuberculosis

C. Rhinosporidium seeberi

D. Treponema pallidum

Clinical presentation and image are indicative of rhinosporidiosis.

Let's discuss the options:

Option	*Statement*	*Remarks*
a	Klebsiella rhinoscleromatis	• It is a gram-negative bacteria which causes rhinoscleroma. • It is also known as Frisch bacillus. • Rhinoscleroma is endemic in north India. • It is also known as woody/Hebra and Tapir nose. • It additionally involves nasopharynx, oropharynx and larynx. • **Biopsy:** Mikulicz cells and Russell bodies are **diagnostic.** • Primary management is medical (Streptomycin, tetracycline etc.).
b	Mycobacterium tuberculosis	• TB of the nose is secondary to pulmonary TB. • It involves the anterior part of nasal septum and anterior end of inferior turbinate. • Hence, it causes perforation in the anterior cartilaginous part of the septum. • **Diagnosis:** Biopsy and AFB stain.
c	Rhinosporidium seeberi	• Rhinosporidium seeberi causes rhinosporidiosis. • Rhinosporidiosis is a chronic granulomatous disease, characterized by large friable polyps in the nose (**most** common site), conjunctiva and occasionally in ears, larynx, bronchus and genitalia. • Stagnant water is the **main** source of infection. Fungal spores are inhaled while taking bath in contaminated ponds and rivers.

Contd.

		• Rhinosporidiosis is **common** in tropical countries, especially in Sri Lanka and India (Tamilnadu, Kerala, Orissa and Andhra Pradesh). • Diagnosis is made by histopathology of the polyps that demonstrates spherules (large sporangia up to 350 µm in size, that contain numerous endospores, each 6-9 µm in size). • Rhinosporidium seeberi has **not** been cultivated yet.
d	Treponema pallidum	• Both congenital and acquired syphilis can be seen in the nose. • Congenital syphilis either presents early (3 weeks to 3 months) after birth as snuffles (catarrhal rhinitis) or late as gummas (solitary lesions showing granulomatous inflammation). • Acquired syphilis may present in primary, secondary or tertiary stage. • In primary stage, it presents as chancre (painless, non-tender, indurated ulcer) of nasal vestibule. • In secondary stage, it presents as mucous patches and snail track ulcers. • **Most** common syphilis seen in the nose is tertiary syphilis. Here gummas are seen on nasal septum. Later on perforations occur in both bony (**more** commonly) and cartilaginous part of septum and hard palate. Saddling of nose may result.

Coming back to the question:

- *Rhinosporidiosis is caused by Rhinosporidium seeberi.*

14. Which of the following option is associated with the causative agent of the clinical condition shown in the image below?

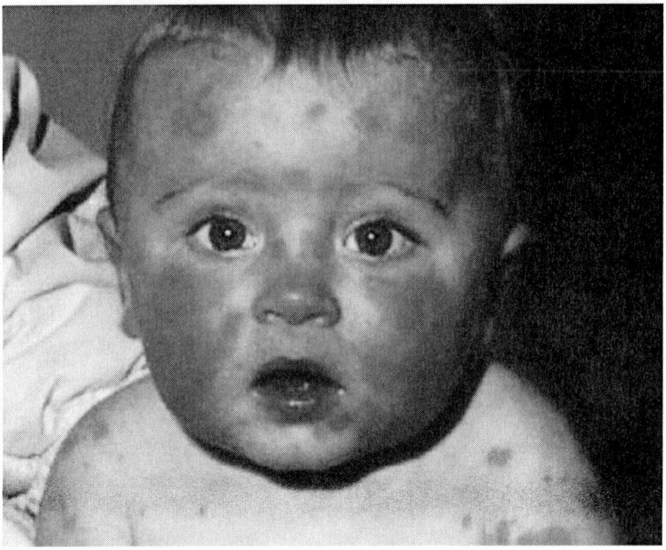

A. Pure red cell aplasia
B. Kaposi sarcoma
C. Molluscum contagiosum
D. Condyloma acuminatum

Image is indicative of erythema infectiosum/fifth disease (shows slapped cheek appearance), which is caused by Parvovirus B-19.

Let's discuss the options:

Option	*Statement*	*Remarks*
a	Pure red cell aplasia	• It can occur in those with underlying immunosuppression due to persistent **Parvovirus B-19** infections, resulting in chronic anemia. • Antibody: IgM (-/+), IgG (-/+). • Real time PCR: $>10^6$ DNA copies/mL.
b	Kaposi sarcoma	• Kaposi sarcoma is seen in clinical stage 4 of HIV/AIDS infection (WHO clinical staging of HIV/AIDS for adults).

Contd.

		• The skin, mouth, hard palate, penis and lower limbs are **common** sites. • It consists of multiple vascular nodules (vascular origin). • Size of the lesion varies from few mms to few cm. • The colour of the lesion is reddish brown or purple. • It **never** involves brain.
c	Molluscum contagiosum	• Molluscum contagiosum virus is an obligate human poxvirus that produces characteristic skin lesions known as molluscum contagiosum. • It produces pink pearly wart-like lesions (2-5 mm in size), umbilicated, with a **characteristic** dimple at the center. • Molluscum bodies are the intracytoplasmic eosinophilic inclusions seen in skin scrapings stained with histopathological stains.
d	Condyloma acuminatum	• Anogenital warts/Condyloma acuminatum is a sexually transmitted disease seen among adults. • It has **low** malignant potential. • It is caused by HPV types 6, 11.

Coming back to the question:

- *Erythema infectiosum and pure red cell aplasia, both are caused by Parvovirus B-19.*

15. A patient undergoes a lung resection surgery for some lung pathology. He was on glucocorticoids therapy for long. Gross specimen of the lung and histopathological staining is shown below. Most likely diagnosis:

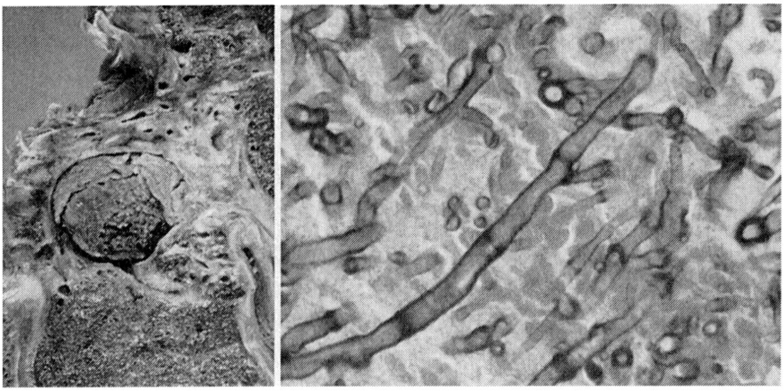

A. Mucormycosis
B. Blastomycosis
C. Candidiasis
D. Aspergillosis

Clinical presentation and image are indicative of pulmonary aspergillosis.

Let's discuss the options:

Option	*Statement*	*Remarks*
a	Mucormycosis	• Agents of mucormycosis require iron as growth factor. Hence conditions with increased iron load are at **higher** risk of developing invasive mucormycosis like diabetic ketoacidosis (**most** important risk factor), end stage renal disease, patients on iron therapy/ Desferroxamine and defects in phagocytic function (neutropenia or steroid therapy). • Histopathological staining of tissue biopsies shows broad **aseptate** hyaline **hyphae** with **wide** angle branching ($>90^{0}$).
b	Blastomycosis	• Blastomycosis is a fungal infection of humans and other animals, notably dogs and cats, caused by the dimorphic fungus, Blastomyces dermatidis.

Contd.

		• Acute pulmonary blastomycosis is the **most** common form. • Skin involvement is the **most** common extrapulmonary form; characterized by either verrucous (**more** common) or ulcerative type of skin lesions. • Histopathological staining of the tissue biopsy specimens reveals thick-walled round yeast cells of 8-15 μm size with single broad-based budding (**figure** of 8 apperance).
c	Candidiasis	• Predisposing factors that are associated with increased risk of infection with *Candida* include extremes of age, patients on steroid/immunosuppressive drugs, post-transplantation, malignancy, HIV infected people, diabetic patients etc. • **Direct microscopy:** Gram staining reveals gram-positive **oval** budding yeast cells with **pseudo-hyphae**.
d	Aspergillosis	• Risk factors for invasive aspergillosis are: **Glucocorticoid** use (most important risk factor), profound neutropenia, neutrophil dysfunction etc. • Pulmonary aspergillosis is the **most** common form of aspergillosis. • **Direct examination:** 10% KOH mount or histological staining of specimens reveals characteristic narrow **septate** hyaline **hyphae** with **acute** angle branching ($<45^{o}$).

Coming back to the question:

- *Aspergillus infection is commonly seen in patients on prolonged steroid therapy and shows narrow septate hyphae with acute angle branching.*

16. Agglutination test is negative till 1:40 but becomes positive with serial dilution. This happens because of:

Tube No.	1	2	3	4	5	6	–
Saline (ml)	1.9	1	1	1	1	1	–
Serum (ml)	0.1	–	–	–	–	–	–
	1 ml→	1 ml→	1ml→	1ml →	1 ml→	1 ml →	1 ml discard
Dilutions	1/20	1/40	1/80	1/160	1/320	1/640	–

A. Excess antibody
B. Excess antigen
C. Low antibody
D. Low antigen

Key points about Agglutination reaction:

- *When a particulate or insoluble antigen is mixed with its antibody in the presence of electrolytes at a suitable temperature and pH, the particles are clumped or agglutinated.*
- *Agglutination is more sensitive than precipitation test and the clumps are better visualized and interpreted than bands or floccules. Hence, agglutination tests are widely used even in today's modern era of diagnosis.*
- *Agglutination reactions are classified as direct, indirect (passive) and reverse passive agglutination reactions.*
- *All these agglutination tests are performed either on a slide, or in tube or in card or some time in microtiter plates.*
- *Tube agglutination:*
    - o *This is a quantitative test done for estimating antibody in serum.*
    - o *The antibody titer can be estimated as the highest dilution of the serum which produces a visible agglutination.*
    - o *Tube agglutination is routinely used for the serological diagnosis of various diseases, such as typhoid fever (Widal test), acute brucellosis, typhus fever (Weil-Felix reaction), infectious mononucleosis (Paul Bunnell test) etc.*
- *Two* ***main*** *problems pertaining to agglutination are prozone phenomenon and blocking antibody; both can cause* ***false****-negative agglutination test.*

- *Prozone phenomenon:*
  - *It is observed that when the concentration of antibody is high (i.e., lower dilutions), there is no agglutination and then, as the sample is diluted, agglutination occurs.*
  - *Lack of agglutination in the prozone is due to* ***antibody excess*** *resulting in very small complexes that do not clump to form visible agglutination.*
  - *This can be obviated by serial dilution of the serum and testing the antigen with each dilution of the serum sample.*

Coming back to the question:

- *Excess antibody in serum may produce a negative agglutination test initially, which can be obviated by serial dilution of the serum.*

PHARMACOLOGY

1. Cyclosporine induced cholestasis is mediated through interference with which of the following protein?

A. MDR1
B. MRP2
C. MDR3
D. BSEP

Key points about iDILI:

- *Idiosyncratic Drug-Induced Liver Injury accounts for more than 40% of hepatitis cases in adults over 50 years and more than 50% of acute fulminant hepatic failure cases.*
- *In addition, approximately 30% of iDILI are cholestatic (drug-induced cholestasis/DIC).*
- *The liver's metabolism and clearance of lipophilic drugs depend on their emission into the bile.*
- *Therefore, many medications cause cholestasis through their interaction with hepatic transporters.*
- *The main canalicular efflux proteins include:*
    - *The bile salt export pump/BSEP protein (ABCB11).*
    - *The multidrug resistance protein-2 (MRP2, ABCC2) regulating the bile salts independent flow by excretion of glutathione.*
    - *The multidrug resistance-1 protein (MDR1, ABCB1) that transport organic cations. The role of this molecule is in driving the excretion of multiple drugs, especially of quaternary cationic amines, converging them into the bile. Drugs interfering with these transporters can lead to an intracellular accumulation of bile/bile constituents, potentially harmful accumulation, and the development of cholestatic liver cell damage. Xenobiotics, cytotoxins, cyclosporine, erythromycin, chlorpromazine, anti-cancer drugs, cardiac glycosides and HIV protease inhibitors.*
    - *The multidrug resistance-3 protein (MDR3, ABCB4).*

Coming back to the question:

- *Cyclosporine induced cholestasis is mediated through interference with MDR-1 protein.*

2. A patient was given Morphine post-surgery for pain relief, after which he developed respiratory depression. Which drug should be used in such a case?

A. Pethidine
B. Atropine
C. Fomepizole
D. Naloxone

Let's discuss the options:

Option	*Statement*	*Remarks*
a	Pethidine	• Pethidine is **primarily** used as an analgesic (substitute of morphine) and in pre-anesthetic medication, but **not** for cough or diarrhoea. • It has also been used to control shivering during recovery from anaesthesia or that attending I.V. infusions. • It is the **preferred** opioid analgesic during labor, because at equianalgesic doses neonatal respiratory depression is **less** marked, but still significant.
b	Atropine	• **Pre-anesthetic medication:** When irritant general anesthetics (ether) were used, prior administration of anticholinergics (atropine) was imperative to check increased salivary and tracheobronchial secretions. • **Peptic ulcer:** Atropinic drugs decrease gastric secretion (fasting and neurogenic phase, but little effect on gastric phase) and afford symptomatic relief in peptic ulcer, though effective doses always produce side effects. • Atropine is used as an antispasmodic, though it is **less** effective in biliary colic and is not able to completely counteract biliary spasm due to opiates (nitrates are more effective). • Atropine ointment (1%) applied 24 hours and 2 hours before is often **preferred** for testing error of refraction in children below 5 years of age.

Contd.

		• Because of its long lasting mydriatic-cycloplegic and local anodyne (pain relieving) action on cornea, atropine is **very** valuable in treatment of iritis, iridocyclitis, choroiditis, keratitis and corneal ulcer. • Atropine is useful in counteracting sinus bradycardia and partial heart block in selected patients where increased vagal tone is responsible, e.g., in some cases of myocardial infarction and in digitalis toxicity. • Atropine is the **specific** antidote for anti-ChE and early mushroom poisoning.
c	Fomepizole	• Fomepizole is the **specific** inhibitor of alcohol dehydrogenase and is the drug of **choice** for methanol poisoning by retarding its metabolism. • It has several advantages over ethanol, viz. longer t½ and lack of inebriating actin, but it is **not** available commercially in India.
d	Naloxone	• Naloxone is the drug of **choice** for morphine poisoning and for reversal of neonatal asphyxia due to opioid use during labor. • It is also used to treat overdose with other opioids and agonist-antagonists (**except** buprenorphine). • It is used to **reverse respiratory depression** due to intraoperative use of opioids • It has also been tried as an adjunct to intraspinal opioid analgesia; reverses respiratory depression without abolishing pain relief.

Coming back to the question:

- *Respiratory depression following morphine use, can be reversed by Naloxone.*

3. A drug was given to a diabetic patient which resulted in improvement in fasting state and post-prandial state blood sugar levels. There was increased GLP-1 induced insulin release and decreased glucagon levels. Which of the following drug was given to the patient?

A. Metformin
B. Alogliptin
C. Pramlintide
D. Liraglutide

Let's discuss the options:

Option	*Statement*	*Remarks*
a	Metformin	• Metformin (Biguanides) do **not** cause insulin release, but presence of insulin is essential for their action. • Metformin is **not** effective in pancreatectomized animals and in type I diabetics. • Metformin suppresses hepatic gluconeogenesis and glucose output from liver. This is the **major** action responsible for lowering of blood glucose in diabetics. • Metformin enhances insulin-mediated glucose uptake and disposal in skeletal muscle and fat. Insulin resistance exhibited in type-2 diabetics is thus overcome. • Interference with mitochondrial respiratory chain and promotes peripheral glucose utilization through anaerobic glycolysis.
b	Alogliptin	• Realizing the key role of DPP-4 in rapid degradation of endogenous GLP-1, orally active inhibitors of this enzyme have been developed as indirectly acting insulin secretagogues. • Alogliptin belongs to DPP-4 inhibitors (Dipeptidyl peptidase-4).

Contd.

c	Pramlintide	• Pramlintide is a synthetic amylin analogue which on S.C. injection before meals attenuates postprandial glycaemia and exerts a centrally mediated anorectic action. • The duration of action is 2-3 hours. • It has been used as an adjunct to meal time insulin injection to suppress the glycaemic peak in both type I and type II diabetics. • Reduction in body weight is an additional benefit.
d	Liraglutide	• GLP-1 (Glucagon-like peptide-1) is an **important** incretin released from the gut in response to ingested glucose. It induces **insulin** release from pancreatic beta cells, inhibits **glucagon** release from alpha cells, slows gastric emptying and suppresses appetite by activating specific GLP-1 receptors, which are cell surface GPCRs. • GLP-1 itself is **not** suitable for clinical use because of rapid degradation by the enzyme dipeptidyl peptidase-4 (DPP-4). • Liraglutide is a recently developed long-acting **GLP-1** agonist and is closely related to the native peptide.

Coming back to the question:

- *Liraglutide promotes GLP-1 mediated insulin release and inhibits glucagon release.*

4. Which of the following drug is used for Trastuzumab-resistant, HER2 positive, advanced breast carcinoma?

A. Erlotinib
B. Vemurafenib
C. Sorafenib
D. Lapatinib

Let's discuss the options:

Option	*Statement*	*Remarks*
a	Erlotinib	• Epidermal growth factor (EGF) receptor is a transmembrane receptor-tyrosine-kinase which regulates growth and differentiation of epithelial cells. • Binding of ligand (EGF) to the extracellular domain of the receptor induces dimerization leading to activation of tyrosine kinase activity of the intracellular domain → autophosphorylation of the kinase and phosphorylation of several cytoplasmic regulatory proteins which modify gene transcription to regulate growth. • Erlotinib is a synthetic compound that penetrates cells, binds to the tyrosine kinase domain of the EGF receptor (also Erbβ_1, or HER1) and **prevents** phosphorylation of regulatory proteins. It acts as EGF receptor inhibitor. • It is found effective in a subtype of non-small cell lung cancer. • It has been combined with gemcitabine for advanced/metastatic pancreatic cancer as well.
b	Vemurafenib	• Vemurafenib is a kinase inhibitor used to treat patients with Erdheim-Chester disease who have the BRAF V600 mutation, and melanoma in patients who have the BRAF V600E mutation.
c	Sorafenib	• Sorafenib is a kinase inhibitor used to treat unresectable liver carcinoma, advanced renal carcinoma, and differentiated thyroid carcinoma.

Contd.

d	Lapatinib	• Lapatinib is used for treatment of solid tumours such as breast and lung cancer. • It is used in patients with advances metastatic breast cancer in conjunction with the chemotherapy drug capecitabine. • Lapatinib is a human epidermal growth factor receptor type 2 (HER2/ ERBB2) tyrosine kinase inhibitor. • It binds to the intracellular phosphorylation domain to prevent receptor autophosphorylation upon ligand binding. • It is indicated in combination with capecitabine for the treatment of patients with advanced or metastatic breast cancer whose tumours overexpress the human epidermal receptor type 2 (**HER2**) protein and who had received prior therapy including an anthracycline (doxorubicin, daunorubicin etc.), a taxane (paclitaxel, estramustine etc.) and **trastuzumab**.

Coming back to the question:

- *Lapatinib is used for HER2 positive advanced breast cancer, which is trastuzumab resistant.*

5. True statement regarding Lithium is:

A. It is not teratogenic
B. It produce fine tremors in therapeutic range blood level
C. It is not absorbed orally
D. It is approved in the management of absence seizures

Let's discuss the options:

Option	*Statement*	*Remarks*
a	It is not teratogenic	• False statement. • Lithium is **contraindicated** during pregnancy; foetal goitre and other congenital abnormalities especially cardiac, can occur; the newborn is often hypotonic.
b	It produce fine tremors in therapeutic range blood level	• **True** statement. • Fine tremors are noted even at therapeutic concentrations of lithium.
c	It is not absorbed orally	• False statement. • Lithium is slowly but well absorbed orally and is **neither** protein bound **nor** metabolized. • It **first** distributes in extracellular water, then gradually enter cells and penetrates into brain, ultimately attaining a rather uniform distribution in total body water.
d	It is approved in the management of absence seizures	• False statement. • Lithium is mainly indicated in controlling acute mania and as prophylaxis in bipolar disorder. • It is **not** used for managing absence seizures. Ethosuximide and valproate are equally efficacious in managing absence seizures, but the latter is **more** commonly used because it would also prevent kindling and emergence of generalized tonic clonic seizures/GTCS.

Coming back to the question:

- *Lithium is teratogenic, absorbed orally, produces fine tremors in therapeutic range blood level but is not used in managing absence seizures.*

6. Which of the following is useful for Vancomycin dosing?

A. Hartford
B. Conventional dosing
C. Online calculator
D. Nomogram

Key points about Nomogram:

- *Nomogram is designed to guide determination of initial empiric dose and interval of intravenous **vancomycin** in hospitalized adults.*
- *In general, the clinical utility of nomograms is limited since it is **not** possible to account for all patient-specific variables.*
- *Use of vancomycin dosing nomograms typically produces steady-state serum concentrations within the targeted range in approximately 44 to 76 percent of patients.*
- *Ideally, the approach to vancomycin dosing approach at a particular institution should be guided by a nomogram developed and validated at that institution, to best reflect the regional patient population.*

		eGFR (mL/min/1.73 m²)		
		> 79	**40-79**	**20-39**
Weight (kg)	**40-59**	750 mg every 12 hours	750 mg every 24 hours	750 mg every 48 hours
	60-74	1000 mg every 12 hours	1000 mg every 24 hours	1000 mg every 48 hours
	75-89	1250 mg every 12 hours	1250 mg every 24 hours	1250 mg every 48 hours
	90-110	1500 mg every 12 hours	1500 mg every 24 hours	1500 mg every 48 hours
	111-125	1750 mg every 12 hours	1750 mg every 24 hours	1750 mg every 48 hours
	> 125	2000 mg every 12 hours	2000 mg every 24 hours	2000 mg every 48 hours

Coming back to the question:

- *Nomogram is helpful in determining initial dose and interval of vancomycin administration.*

7. A known case of mood disorder was started on some drug but during the course of treatment, he developed priapism. Most likely drug is:

A. Bupropion
B. Venlafaxine
C. Trazodone
D. Mirtazapine

Let's discuss the options:

Option	*Statement*	*Remarks*
a	Bupropion	• This inhibitor of dopamine/DA and noradrenaline/NA uptake has excitant rather than sedative property. • It is metabolized into an amphetamine like compound which can cause presynaptic release of DA and NA. • A sustained-release formulation is marketed as an aid to smoking cessation. • Better results are obtained when it is combined with nicotine patch. • The nicotine withdrawal symptoms were **less** severe in bupropion recipients. • However, long-term efficacy is unknown, and it can cause insomnia, agitation, dry mouth and nausea, but **not** sexual side-effects. • Seizures occur in overdose and in predisposed patients due to lowering of seizure threshold.
b	Venlafaxine	• A novel antidepressant, referred to as SNRI (serotonin and noradrenaline reuptake inhibitor), because it inhibits uptake of both NA and 5-HT but, in contrast to older TCAs, does not

Contd.

		interact with cholinergic, adrenergic or histaminergic receptors or have sedative property. • It does **not** produce the usual side effects of TCAs; tends to raise **rather** than depress BP and is safer in overdose. • Prominent side-effects are nausea, sweating, anxiety, dizziness, impotence and withdrawal reactions on discontinuation.
c	Trazodone	• It is the **first** atypical antidepressant; **less** efficiently blocks 5-HT uptake and has prominent α adrenergic and weak 5-HT_2 antagonist action. • The latter may contribute to its antidepressant effect, which nevertheless is modest. • It is sedative but **not** anticholinergic, causes bradycardia rather than tachycardia, does **not** interfere with intracardiac conduction – **less** prone to cause arrhythmia and better suited for elderly. • Inappropriate, prolonged and painful penile erection **(priapism)** occurs in few recipients resulting in impotence in a fraction of these. • The α_1 adrenergic blocking property has been held responsible for this effect as well as for postural hypotension.
d	Mirtazapine	• This antidepressant acts by a novel mechanism, viz. blocks α_2 auto- (on NA neurones) and hetero- (on 5-HT neurones) receptors enhancing both NA and 5-HT release. • It is a H_1 blocker and quite sedative, but **not** anticholinergic or antidopaminergic.

Contd.

		• Increased appetite and weight gain is frequent. • Sexual dysfunction is **not** a problem with mirtazapine.

Coming back to the question:

- *Priapism is a side-effect of Trazodone.*

8. All of the following factors are responsible for teratogenicity due to Thalidomide EXCEPT:

A. Cereblon binding
B. Inhibition of IL-2, IL-4 and IL-5
C. Suppression of angiogenesis
D. Reactive oxygen species mediated cell damage

Key points about mechanism of action, underlying Thalidomide embryopathy:

- *Cereblon binding:*
  - o *The thalidomide binding target, Cereblon, an ubiquitin ligase, which if prevented from binding can reduce thalidomide induced damage in embryos.*
  - o *Thalidomide is thought to initiate teratogenesis by binding Cereblon, which presumably prevents Cereblon from establishing the E3 ubiquination complex to target molecules for removal causing misregulation of developmental signalling molecules.*
- *Suppression of angiogenesis:*
  - o *Thalidomide's antiangiogenic actions – the drug's ability to induce cell death and generate reactive oxygen species.*
  - o *Blood vessels are essential for normal embryonic development.*
  - o *Blood vessels supply oxygen and nutrients to growing tissues and remove unwanted waste products.*
  - o *During embryogenesis, vessels form firs by vasculogenesis and are then modified into the complex vascular tree for embryonic and fetal and throughout adult life by angiogenesis.*

- o *Blood vessels are essential for normal embryonic development, and vessel loss or disruption can unsurprisingly result in death or birth defect.*
- *Another attractive hypothesis suggests Thalidomide can induce formation of reactive oxygen species/**ROS**, which causes oxidative stress to cells, which has been proposed to cause limb defects.*

Coming back to the question:

- *Factors responsible for teratogenicity of Thalidomide are Cereblon binding, suppression of angiogenesis and reactive oxygen species mediated cell damage.*

9. Osimertinib is beneficial in Non-small cell lung carcinoma arising due to:

A. L-858R mutation
B. T-790M mutation
C. M-790T mutation
D. T-890M mutation

Key points about Osimertinib:

- *Osimertinib is used to treat locally advanced or metastatic non-small cell lung cancer (**NSCLC**), if the cancer cells are positive for the **T790M** mutation in the gene coding for EGFR or for the activating EGFR mutations.*
- *The T790M mutation may be de novo or acquired following first-line treatment with other EGFR tyrosine kinase inhibitors, such as geftinib, erlotinib and afatinib.*
- *In the US, EGFR exon 19 deletions, exon 21 L858R mutations or the T790M status of the patient prior to the treatment with Osimertinib must be detected.*
- *In people treated with Osimertinib, resistance usually develops within approximately 10 months.*
- *Resistance mediated by an exon 20 C797S mutation accounts for the majority of resistance cases.*
- *It can cause fetal harm, so should not be used in women who are pregnant, and women who take it should avoid becoming pregnant.*
- *Caution should be taken in people with a history of interstitial lung disease, since the drug can cause severe ILD or pneumonitis.*
- *Caution should also be taken in people with a predisposition to long QT syndrome as the drug can provoke this.*

Coming back to the question:

- *Osimertinib is used to treat non-small cell lung cancer arising due to T790M mutation.*

10. KEYNOTE-189 clinical trial studied the:

A. Efficacy of Pembrolizumab plus chemotherapy in non-small cell lung carcinoma
B. Efficacy of Ipilimumab in non-small cell lung carcinoma
C. Efficacy of Nivolumab plus chemotherapy in non-small cell lung carcinoma
D. Efficacy of Atezolizumab is in non-small cell lung carcinoma

Key points about trials related to treatment of NSCLC:

- *Multiple phase 3 clinical trials using immunotherapy in the first line of treatment of non-small cell lung cancer (NSCLC) were published.*
- ***Pembrolizumab** in KEYNOTE-024, KEYNOTE-042, **KEYNOTE-189** and KEYNOTE-407.*
- *In KEYNOTE-189, first line Pembrolizumab plus Pemetrexed-Platinum significantly improved overall survival and progression free survival compared with Placebo plus Pemetrexed-Platinum in patients with metastatic NSCLC, irrespective of tumour programmed death-ligand 1 (PD-L1) expression.*
- *Nivolumab and Ipilimumab in CHECKMATE-227 and CHECKMATE 9LA.*
- *Atezolizumab in IMpower110, IMpower130 and IMpower150.*
- *NSCLC cells expressing programmed death-ligand 1 (PD-L1), could interact with programmed death receptor 1 (PD-1) expressed on the surface of T cells, and result in decreased tumour cell kill by the immune system.*
- *Pembrolizumab and Nivolumab are anti PD-1 monoclonal antibodies.*
- *Ipilimumab is a monoclonal antibody that targets Cytotoxic T-lymphocyte-associated protein 4 (CTLA-4) on the surface of T cells.*
- *Atezolizumab is an anti PD-L1 monoclonal antibody.*

Coming back to the question:

- *KEYNOTE-189 clinical trial evaluated the efficacy of Pembrolizumab + Pemetrexed-Platinum versus Placebo + Pemetrexed-Platinum in NSCLC.*

11. Which of the following is a rare but severe side-effect of Clozapine that requires regular monitoring?

A. Suicidal tendencies
B. Myocarditis
C. Agranulocytosis
D. Intracerebral bleeding

Key points about Clozapine:

- *Clozapine is the **first** atypical antipsychotic; pharmacologically distinct from CPZ (Chlorpromazine) and related drugs in that:*
  - o *It has only weak Dopaminergic-2 (D2) blocking action.*
  - o *It produces few/**no** extrapyramidal symptoms.*
  - o *Tardive dyskinesia is **rare.***
  - o *Prolactin level do **not** rise.*
- *Both positive and negative symptoms of schizophrenia are improved and clozapine is the **most** effective drug in refractory schizophrenia, i.e., patients not responding to typical neuroleptics may respond to it.*
- *Its major limitation is **higher** incidence of **agranulocytosis** (0.8%) and other blood dyscrasias: weekly **monitoring** of leucocyte count is required.*
- *Metabolic complication like weight gain, hyperlipidemia and precipitation of diabetes is another **major** limitation.*
- *High dose can induce seizures even in non-epileptics.*
- *Other side effects are sedation, unstable BP, tachycardia and urinary incontinence.*
- *Few cases of myocarditis have been reported which start like flu but may progress to death.*
- *Clozapine is used as a reserve drug in refractory schizophrenia.*

Coming back to the question:

- *Agranulocytosis is a complication of Clozapine, which requires weekly monitoring of leucocyte count.*

12. Match the following:

Drug	*Adrenergic receptors*
1. Mirabegron	**A. Beta-2**
2. Indacaterol	**B. Beta-3**
3. Betaxolol	**C. Beta**
4. Isoproterenol	**D. Beta-1**

Lead – Choose the best answer from the codes given below:

A. 1-B, 2-A, 3-D, 4-C
B. 1-C, 2-B, 3-A, 4-D
C. 1-A, 2-B, 3-C, 4-D
D. 1-C, 2-A, 3-B, 4-D

Let's discuss the options:

Option	*Statement*	*Remarks*
1	Mirabegron	• Mirabegron is a **beta-3** adrenergic agonist. • It is used in the management of overactive bladder. • It works by relaxing the bladder muscles to prevent urgent, frequent, or uncontrolled urination.
2	Indacaterol	• Indacaterol is an inhaled long-acting **beta-2** adrenergic agonist. • It is used to relax bronchial smooth muscle and improve symptoms and airflow obstruction caused by COPD and moderate to severe asthma.
3	Betaxolol	• Betaxolol is a **beta-1** selective blocker offering the **advantage** of less bronchopulmonary and probably less cardiac, central and metabolic side effects. • In addition, it appears to exert a protective effect on retinal neurones independent of intraocular tension lowering, by blocking some Ca^{2+} channels and reducing Na^+/Ca^{2+} influx.

Contd.

4	Isoproterenol	• Isoprenaline/Isoproterenol has **beta-1** + **beta-2** + **beta-3** adrenergic agonist action, but **no** alpha receptor action. • It is occasionally used to maintain idioventricular rate till the pacemaker is implanted. • For bronchial asthma, it has been superseded by selective beta-2 agonists.

Coming back to the question:

Drug	*Adrenergic receptors*
1. Mirabegron	*B. Beta-3*
2. Indacaterol	*A. Beta-2*
3. Betaxolol	*D. Beta-1*
4. Isoproterenol	*C. Beta*

13. Which of the following is a new drug approved by FDA in the management of Rett's syndrome?

A. Ubrogepant
B. Lasmiditan
C. Trofinetide
D. Sparsentan

Let's discuss the options:

Option	*Statement*	*Remarks*
a	Ubrogepant	• Ubrogepant is indicated for the acute treatment of migraine headaches with or without aura in adults. • It is the **first** oral calcitonin gene-related peptide (CGRP) receptor antagonist approved for the treatment of migraine.
b	Lasmiditan	• Lasmiditan is a **highly** selective agonist of $5\text{-}HT_{1F}$ receptors, carrying virtually no affinity for other receptors, which appear to be largely responsible for the adverse effect profile of its predecessors – in other words, Lasmiditan's selectivity allows for the successful termination of migraines without causing vasoconstriction.

Contd.

		• Triptans (Sumatriptan) abort migraine via action at several serotonin receptors, including 5-HT_{1D} and 5-HT_{1B} receptors, and activity at the 5-HT_{1B} receptor has been specifically implicated in their vasoconstrictive activity. • Selectively for 5-HT_{1F}, a lack of vasoconstrictive activity, and the ability to terminate migraines through neuronal inhibition has resulted in the creation of a new class of anti-migraine medications in which Lasmiditan is the first and **only** member; the neutrally-acting anti-migraine medications (NAAMAs).
c	Trofinetide	• Trofinetide is a synthetic analogue of glycine-proline-glutamate, the N-terminal tripeptide of the insulin-like growth factor 1 protein, and has demonstrated clinical benefit in phase 2 studies in **Rett** syndrome. • Trofinetide is believed to work by reducing inflammation and apoptosis of neurons in Rett syndrome. • Rett syndrome is a rare, genetic neurodevelopmental disorder. • It is characterized by loss of verbal communication with limited nonverbal skills, loss of fine and gross motor function (including purposeful hand use), behavioural issues, seizures, hand stereotypies and gastrointestinal problems.
d	Sparsentan	• Sparsentan is an endothelin and angiotensin II receptor antagonist indicated to reduce proteinuria in adults with primary IgA nephropathy at risk of rapid disease progression.

Coming back to the question:

- *Trofinetide is useful in Rett syndrome.*

14. Which of the following is true regarding therapeutic index of a drug?

A. Denotes safety and efficacy in an individual
B. Denotes safety and efficacy in population
C. Ratio of median lethal dose in 50% of animals to median effective dose in 50% of animals
D. Ratio of median effective dose in 50% of animals to median lethal dose in 50% of animals

Key points about Therapeutic index:

- *The gap between the therapeutic effect Dose Response Curve/DRC and the adverse effect DRC defines the safety margin/therapeutic index of a drug.*
- *In experimental animals, therapeutic index is often calculated as:*
    - o *Medial toxic/**lethal** dose.*
    - o *Median **effective**/therapeutic dose.*
- *Where: Median effective dose (ED_{50}) is the dose which produces the specified effect in 50% individuals and median toxic dose (TD_{50})/median lethal dose (LD_{50}) is the dose which kills 50% of the recipients.*

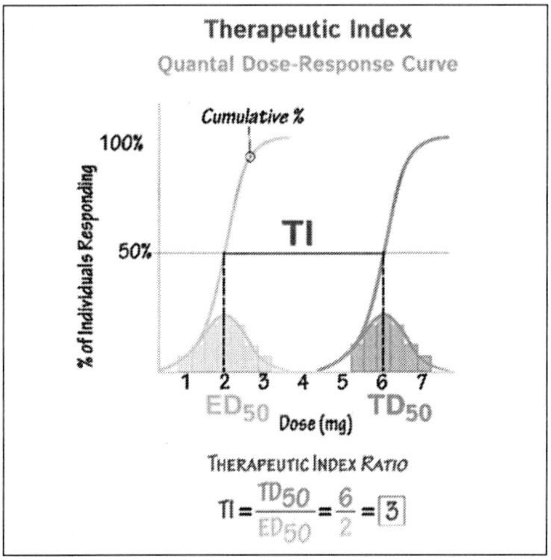

Coming back to the question:

- *Therapeutic index is the ratio of median lethal dose to median effective dose.*

15. A known case of type-II DM was started on some drug. This drug decreased her HbA_{1c} from 7.6% to 6.8% but she developed itching near vulvovaginal area. The drug in discussion is:

A. Linagliptin
B. Acarbose
C. Canagliflozin
D. Pioglitazone

Let's discuss the options:

Option	*Statement*	*Remarks*
a	Linagliptin	• Realizing the key role of DPP-4 in rapid degradation of endogenous GLP-1, orally active inhibitors of this enzyme have been developed as indirectly acting insulin secretagogues. • Linagliptin belongs to DPP-4 inhibitors (Dipeptidyl peptidase-4).
b	Acarbose	• Acarbose is a complex oligosaccharide which reversibly inhibits α-glucosidases, the final enzymes for the digestion of carbohydrates in brush border of small intestine mucosa. • It slows down and decreases digestion and absorption of polysaccharides (starch etc.) and sucrose. • In addition, GLP-1 (Glucagon-like peptide-1) release is promoted, which may contribute to the effect. • Regular use lowers HbA_{1c} modestly (by 0.4 – 0.8%), but change in body weight and lipid levels is minimal. • Flatulence, abdominal discomfort and loose stools are produced in about 50% patients due to fermentation of unabsorbed carbohydrates.

Contd.

		• Patient acceptability is poor due to gastrointestinal symptoms.
c	Canagliflozin	• Canagliflozin is a sodium-glucose co-transporter 2 (SGLT2) inhibitor used to manage hyperglycemia in type 2 diabetes mellitus. • The SGLT2 is found in the proximal tubules of the kidney, and reabsorbs filtered glucose form the renal tubular lumen. • Canagliflozin inhibits the SGLT2 co-transporter. • This inhibition leads to lower reabsorption of filtered glucose into the body and decreases the renal threshold for glucose (RTG), leading to increased glucose excretion in the urine. • Canagliflozin decreases **HbA_{1c}** levels by 0.77% to 1.16% when given by itself, in combination with metformin, in combination with metformin and a sulfonylurea, in combination with metformin and pioglitazone, or in combination with insulin, from initial HbA_{1c} levels of 7.8 – 8.1% • Canagliflozin is associated with increased incidence of urinary tract infections, **fungal** infections of the genital area, thirst, elevation in LDL cholesterol, increased urination and episodes of low BP. • Rarely, use of Canagliflozin is associated with necrotizing fasciitis of the perineum (Fournier gangrene).
d	Pioglitazone	• Only one thiazolidinedione Pioglitazone is currently available. • This class of oral antidiabetic drugs are selective agonist for the nuclear

Contd.

		peroxisome proliferator-activated receptor γ (PPARγ) which is expressed mainly in fat cells, but also in muscle and some other cells. • It enhances the transcription of several insulin responsive genes. • Glitazones tend to reverse insulin resistance by enhancing GLUT4 expression and translocation. • Entry of glucose into muscle and fat is improved. • Hepatic gluconeogenesis is also suppressed. • Pioglitazone is well tolerated; adverse effects are plasma volume expansion, edema, weight gain, headache, myalgia and mild anemia. • Few cases of hepatic dysfunction have been reported; CHF may be precipitated or worsened. • Monitoring of liver function is advised.

Coming back to the question:

- *Canagliflozin reduces HbA_{1c} in type 2 DM by 1% but can cause fungal infections of genital area, which can present as itching in vulvovaginal area.*

FORENSIC MEDICINE

1. All of the following are correct regarding postmortem changes EXCEPT:

A. Cadaveric spasm is seen only in one group of muscles
B. Adipocere formation can be seen in drowning case
C. Greenish discoloration can be seen in the skin of infrahepatic area in putrefaction
D. In drowning cases, postmortem staining is seen over the entire limbs

Let's discuss the options:

Option	*Statement*	*Remarks*
a	Cadaveric spasm is seen only in one group of muscles	• True statement. • Cadaveric spasm (cataleptic rigidity) is a rare condition. • In this, the muscles that were contracted during life become stiff and rigid immediately after death without passing into the stage of primary relaxation. • As such, the change preserves the exact attitude of the person at the time of death for several hours afterwards. • This is usually limited to a **single** group of voluntary muscles and frequently involves the hands. • Occasionally, the whole body is affected as seen in soldiers shot in battle, when the body may retain the posture which is assumed at the moment of death.

Contd.

b	Adipocere formation can be seen in drowning case	• True statement. • Adipocere is a modification of putrefaction. • In this, the fatty tissues of the body change into a substance known as adipocere. • It is seen most commonly in bodies immersed in water or in damp, warm environment. • A warm, moist, anaerobic environment favours adipocere formation. • It is more frequently seen in females, the well-nourished mature newborn children, the obese and in corpses that have been **submerged** in water for a long period. • Water helps to remove glycerine which is formed during hydrolysis of the fats. • The water required for the hydrolysis is obtained mainly from the body tissues, which therefore become more and more dehydrated. • In a body immersed in water, this fluid contributes to the hydrolysis of the subcutaneous fats.
c	Greenish discoloration can be seen in the skin of infra-hepatic area in putrefaction	• True statement. • The disintegration of body tissues after death is known as decomposition. • The terms decomposition and putrefaction are used as synonyms. • The first external sign of putrefaction in a body lying in air is usually a **greenish** discoloration of the skin over the region of the caecum,

Contd.

		which lies fairly superficially, and where the contents of the bowel are more fluid and full of bacteria. • The colour results from the conversion of hemoglobin of blood into sulfmethemoglobin by the hydrogen sulphide formed in the large intestine and escaping into the surrounding tissues.
d	In drowning cases, postmortem staining is seen over the entire limbs	• False statement. • Postmortem staining hypostasis is the bluish-purple or purplish-red (due to deoxyhemoglobin) discoloration, which appears under the skin in the most superficial layers of the dermis (rete mucosum) of the dependent parts of the body after death, due to capillovenous distension. • In drowning, postmortem staining is usually found on the face, the upper part of the chest, hands, lower arms, feet and the calves, as they are the dependent parts.

Coming back to the question:

- *In drowning cases, postmortem staining is not seen over the entire limbs. In limbs, it is limited to hands and lower arms and feet and calves, as these are the dependent parts.*

2. A young male had been brought by the police in a drunken state. Smell of alcohol was coming from his mouth. There was conjunctival redness. He was able to walk in a straight line and all his motor functions were also normal. He was conscious and he can talk normally. As a medical officer, what will be your opinion?

A. He had not consumed any alcohol at all
B. He had taken alcohol but is not under any influence

C. He had taken alcohol and is under full influence

D. He had taken alcohol and is under full influence but is not creating any nuisance

Key points about Alcohol poisoning:

- *Stage of excitement:*
  - o *There is **first** a feeling of well-being and a certain slight excitation.*
  - o *The actions, speech and emotions are **less** restrained due to lowering of the inhibition normally exercised by the higher centres of the brain.*
  - o *There is increased confidence and a **lack** of self-control, which is a **constant** feature of alcohol poisoning.*
  - o *The person may disclose secrets.*
  - o *Normal good manners are forgotten.*
  - o *At blood concentration of 30 mg%, impairment of cognitive function, motor coordination and sensory perception occur.*
- *Stage of incoordination:*
  - o *When the alcohol content of blood attains a level of 150-250 mg/100 ml, the sense perception and skilled movements are affected.*
  - o *The increased loss of the inhibitory action of the higher centres causes an alteration in the conduct of the individual.*
  - o *He may become carefree, cheerful, ill-tempered, irritable, excitable, quarrelsome, sleepy, and so on, according to the dominant impulses which have been released.*
  - o *There is certain clumsiness and incoordination in the fine and more skilled movements, as shown by slight alteration in speech and in the fine finger movements.*
  - o *The breath smells of alcohol.*
  - o *The face is flushed and the pulse is rapid.*
- *Stage of coma:*
  - o *In this stage, the motor and sensory cells are deeply affected, speech becomes thick and slurring, coordination is markedly affected, causing the patient to become giddy, stagger and possibly to fall.*
  - o *The person passes into a state of coma with stertorous breathing.*

Coming back to the question:

- *If a person, is able to walk in a straight line, if his motor functions are normal, if he is conscious and if he can talk normally even after consuming alcohol, we can say that he had taken alcohol, but he is not under any influence of alcohol.*

3. Which of the following poison is associated with blackfoot disease?

A. Copper B. Cadmium

C. Arsenic D. Antimony

Key points about Blackfoot disease:

- *Blackfoot disease, a unique peripheral arterial disease characterized by severe systemic arteriosclerosis, as well as dry gangrene and spontaneous amputations of affected extremities and end stages, has been well documented as a characteristic vascular disease associated with long-term* ***arsenic*** *exposure.*
- *Diagnostic criteria for Blackfoot disease include objective signs of ischemia (i.e., absence of arterial pulsations, pallor on elevation, or rubor on dependency of ischemic extremities) and various degrees of ischemic changes in the skin, as well as subjective symptoms of ischemia (i.e., intermittent claudication, pain at rest, and ischemic neuropathy).*
- *Extensive pathological study showed that 30% of Blackfoot disease patients had histological lesions compatible with thromboangiitis obliterans, and 70% showed changes of arteriosclerosis obliterans.*

Let's discuss the options:

Option	*Statement*	*Remarks*
a	Copper	• Chronic poisoning may occur in workers with metal due to inhalation of dust or from food being contaminated with verdigris. • Chronic inhalation of copper sulphate spray can cause vineyard's sprayer's lung disease characterised by a histiocytic granulomatous lung.

Contd.

		• Symptoms consists of gradual anemia, **green** line on gums, colic, peripheral neuritis, atrophy of muscles etc.
b	Cadmium	• Cadmium poisoning causes proteinuria and painful bone lesions known as Ouch-Ouch disease.
c	Arsenic	• Gastroenteric type is the **most** common form of acute poisoning of arsenic, and **resembles** bacterial food poisoning. • Initially the stools are dark-coloured, stinking and bloody, but later becomes colourless, odourless and watery resembling **rice**-water stools of cholera. A **garlicky** odour of breath and faeces may be noted. • Skin changes in chronic poisoning include raindrop type skin pigmentation (pigmentation consists of a finely mottled brown change mostly on the skin flexures, temples, eyelids and neck), rash (**resembling** fading measles rash), Aldrich-Mees lines (transverse white lines in the fingernails).
d	Antimony	• Metallic antimony is not poisonous. • Antimony potassium tartrate (tartar emetic), occurs in the form of whitish or whitish-yellow powder, and antimony trichloride (butter of antimony) are poisonous. • The mode of action and symptoms of acute and chronic antimony poisoning are **similar** to arsenic poisoning.

Coming back to the question:

- *Blackfoot disease is associated with long-term arsenic exposure.*

4. A 5 years old child went to the temple with his grandmother and something bite him. He started crying inconsolable due to burning sensation at the site of bite and was taken to nearby hospital. Examination revealed altered sensorium, lacrimation, increased drooling of saliva, increased sweating, cold clammy skin, pallor and prolonged priapism. His vitals were: BP – 148/93 mm Hg, Heart rate – 153/minute, respiratory rate – 38/minute and sPO$_2$ – 96%. Which of the following should be used in managing such a case?

A. Methylprednisolone B. Epinephrine
C. Prazosin D. Anti-venom

Clinical presentation is indicative of scorpion sting.

Key points about Scorpion sting:

- *The venom of scorpion is clear, colourless toxalbumin, and can be classified as either hemolytic or neurotoxic.*
- *Its toxicity is more than that of snakes, but **only** a small quantity is injected.*
- *The venom is potent autonomic stimulator resulting in the release of massive amounts of catecholamines from the adrenals.*
- *Scorpion bite delays the inactivation of sodium channels of autonomic nervous system resulting in autonomic storm.*
- *The scorpion venom acts as a powerful stimulus for massive release of catecholamines, suppression of insulin secretion, and elevation of plasma angiotensin II level, which in turn cause pathological changes, metabolic disturbances, and cardiovascular manifestations of scorpion sting.*
- *Signs and symptoms:*
    - o *Site of bite is having a red wheal with a hole in the centre and severe **burning** pain radiates from the site.*
    - o *There is feeling of giddiness and fainting.*
    - o *Excessive **sweating** and **salivation**.*
    - o *Death occur in **children** from pulmonary edema and respiratory depression and it is rare in adults.*

Let's discuss the options:

Option	*Statement*	*Remarks*
a, b	Methylprednisolone, Epinephrine	• There is still a great controversy regarding specific drug therapy for scorpion sting and different regimens have been tried so far, such as, steroids, adrenaline, lytic cocktail regimen and many more.
c	Prazosin	• Prazosin has been suggested by some as the ***first*** line drug for the management of severe scorpion envenomation. • Prazosin antagonises the effects of catecholamines thereby preventing further damage of myocardium though it cannot reverse the damage. • Prazosin also acts by reducing the preload, after load and blood pressure without increase in heart rate. • It is an inhibitor of phospho-di-esterase and cause accumulation of cGMP and inhibits formation of inositol phosphate. • Thus, Prazosin results in blunting of catecholamine action on myocardium. • It also increases insulin secretion. • This results in correction of hyperglycemia, hyperkalemia, and helps in saving the myocardial muscle.
d	Antivenom	• Scorpion antivenom, is also available, but its utility in the management of these cases is still doubtful.

Coming back to the question:

- *Prazosin is the first line drug for scorpion sting.*

5. In a case of chronic cocaine poisoning, tactile hallucination of insects crawling under the skin, is known as:

A. Narcolepsy
B. Formication
C. Oneiroid
D. Dipsomania

Let's discuss the options:

Option	***Statement***	***Remarks***
a	Narcolepsy	• Narcolepsy is a sleep disorder that causes an urge to fall asleep suddenly during the daytime that's almost impossible to resist.
b	Formication	• Magnan's symptom/Cocaine bug is characteristic feature of cocainism, in which there is a feeling as if grains of sand are lying under the skin or some small insects are creeping on the skin giving rise to itching sensation (**formication**, tactile hallucination) with resultant excoriation, leading to irregular scratches and ulcers.
c	Oneiroid	• Oneiroid state is a dream-like state, which may last for days or weeks. • The patient suffers from mental confusion, amnesia, illusions, hallucinations, disorientation, agitation and anxiety. • It occurs in delirium and early schizophrenia.
d	Dipsomania	• It is an irresistible desire for alcoholic drinks at periodic intervals.

Coming back to the question:

- *In a case of chronic cocaine poisoning, tactile hallucination of insects crawling under the skin, is known as formication.*

6. A patient of gunshot injury presented with only abrasion collar near the entry wound. What is the possible range of gunshot?

A. Contact shot
B. Close shot
C. Near shot
D. Distant shot

Let's discuss the options:

Option	*Statement*	*Remarks*
a	Contact shot	• **All** the discharge from the muzzle, i.e., gases, flame, powder, smoke and metallic particles are blown into the track taken by the bullet through the body. • Singeing of the hairs may be present due to the escape of hot gases by the sides of the muzzle end.
b	Close shot	• This term is applied when the victim is within the range of the **flame**, i.e., 5 to 8 cm. • The skin is burnt with singeing of the hair. • The skin surrounding the wound is hyperaemic and shows some bruising, burning, blackening and tattooing. • Blackening can be wiped off the skin by a wet cloth, but the tattooing **cannot** be wiped off. • Abraded collar and grease or dirt collar are present.
c	Near shot	• This term is applied when the victim is within the range of **powder** deposition, and outside the range of flame, and smoke, i.e., up to 50 cm. • It is due to absence of flame so there is **no** burning but singeing is present due to hot gases. • Tattooing is also present in these cases.

Contd.

		• The entrance wound is seen as a round hole, slightly smaller than the diameter of the bullet, due to elasticity of the skin, with a bruised and inverted margin and a zone of blackening and tattooing. • Abrasion and grease collar are present.
d	Distant shot	• Above 50 cm. • A shot which is fired from a distance **more** than the range of powder and smoke is considered as distant shot. • The entrance wound is smaller than the missile, due to elasticity of the skin. • Burning, blackening and tattooing are **not** seen. • The skin adjacent to the hole shows two zones, the inner of grease collar and the outer of abraded collar.

Coming back to the question:

- *A distant shot is fired from a distance more than the range of powder and smoke so in such wounds, an inner grease collar and an outer abrasion collar is seen.*

7. A 16 years old girl was brought by police, along with her mother, as an alleged case of rape 2 days back. As a medical officer, what will be your first step, from the given options?

A. Take consent from mother for genital examination
B. Take proper detailed history
C. Start the examination and note down injuries
D. Undress the patient

Key points about Outline of a planned procedure for examination of the rape victim:

- *The victim should be examined when there is a requisition from the investigating police officer or the Magistrate. The victim of rape may go directly to the doctor, who should examine her after obtaining her consent, and after examination he should inform the concerned police station, so that the due legal process can be set in motion.*

- *The written, witnessed consent of the woman for examination, collection of specimens, taking of photographs, treatment, and for release of information to the police, and if she is under 12 years, or of unsound mind, the consent of her parents must be taken in writing.*
- *The victim should be identified by the escorting police constable, whose name and number should be recorded.*
- *The name of the victim and her parent, marital status, residence, occupation, time, date, year, place of examination and by whom requisition is given should be noted.*
- *The victim is examined in the presence of a third person, preferably a female nurse or a female relative of the woman, whose name should be recorded.*
- *The examination should be carried out without delay.*
- *Statements of the victim and of others with her are recorded separately.*
- *Previous history with regard to sexual experience, menses, vaginal discharge, venereal disease etc. should be recorded.*
- *The age should be determined and the height and weight recorded.*
- *The physical development should be noted.*
- *An attempt at undressing the woman should not be made, but she should be requested to undress herself.*
- *If the victim is in menstruation, a second examination should be done after the stoppage of menstruation.*
- *Her general demeanour; emotional and mental state should be observed while she tells her story.*
- *If it appears that she is under the influence of alcohol or drugs, it must be noted and sample of blood, and urine should be collected.*
- *The gait should be observed.*

Coming back to the question:

- *In a case of examination of rape victim, consent should be taken first (by the victim if she is above 12 years of age) followed by detailed history and then medical examination (general physical and anogenital).*

8. Which of the following is NOT a confirmative evidence of ante-mortem drowning?

A. Positive diatom test
B. Water in stomach
C. Washerwoman hands
D. Frothing from nostrils and mouth

Let's discuss the options:

Option	*Statement*	*Remarks*
a	Positive diatom test	• True statement. • Diatoms are microscopic unicellular or colonial algae. • The drowning fluid and the particles in it, e.g., diatoms and planktons, pass from the ruptured alveolar wall into lymph channels and pulmonary veins and thus enter the left heart. • **Only** a live body with a circulation could transport diatoms from the lungs to the brain, bone marrow, liver and other viscera, and skeletal muscle. • The bone marrow is highly suitable and reliable. • The marrow of long bones, such as the femur, tibia and humerus or sternum is examined for diatoms.
b	Water in stomach	• True statement. • The stomach contains water in about 70% of cases of drowning.

Contd.

		• If the chemical and microscopic nature of the water is same as that of the medium of submersion, it is a valuable **confirmatory** evidence of drowning, but it is possible that the victim might have drunk the same water shortly before death. • The small intestine may contain water in about 20% cases. • This sign is regarded as **positive** evidence of death by drowning as it depends on peristaltic movement which is a vital act.
c	Washerwoman hands	• False statement. • Cutis anserina, washerwoman appearance of the palms and soles, pulmonary edema, and hemorrhage into the petrous and mastoid bones can be found in a victim of drug overdose **thrown** in water, and the victim of heart attack collapsing into water.
d	Frothing from nostrils and mouth	• True statement. • A fine, white, lathery froth or foam is seen at the mouth and nostrils, which is one of the most **characteristic** external signs of drowning. • The inhalation of water irritates the mucous membrane of the air-passages due to which the tracheal and bronchial glands secrete large quantities of tenacious mucus, and the alveolar lining cell irritation produces edema fluid.

Coming back to the question:

- *Positive diatom test, presence of water in the stomach and frothing from nostrils and mouth are important evidences of ante-mortem drowning.*

9. What is not included in the RIGHT approach of the guidelines in management of snakebites?

A. Reassurance
B. Incision
C. Go to the hospital
D. Tell the treating doctor about toxicity features

Key points about RIGHT approach in treating snakebites:

- ***R****eassurance.*
- ***I****mmobilization.*
- ***G****etting to the* ***H****ospital.*
- ***T****elling the treating doctor.*

Coming back to the question:

- *'I' in RIGHT approach in treating snakebite cases, is immobilization and not incision.*

10. Identify the condition:

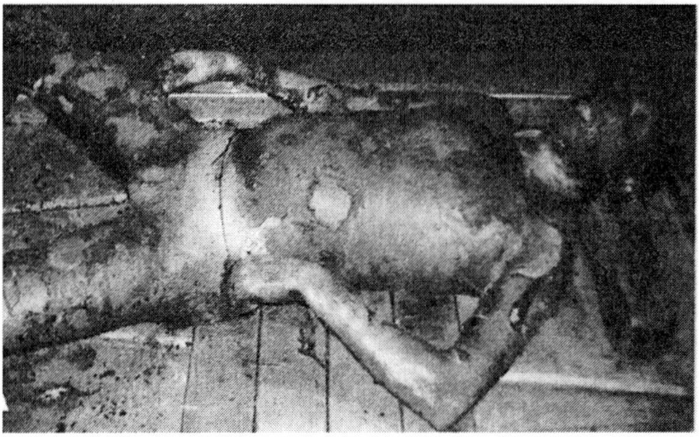

A. Postmortem burns
B. Mummification
C. Antemortem burns
D. High voltage burns

Let's discuss the options:

Option	***Statement***	***Remarks***
a	Postmortem burns	• **Line of redness:** Absent. • **Redness:** Base of blister is dry and yellow; contains air and no protein or chloride but at time traces may be seen; inflammatory reaction is absent. • **Vital reaction:** Negative.
b	Mummification	• It is a modified form of putrefaction and is characterized by drying or shrivelling of the tissue due to dehydration of the body constituents. • The body assumes a dried, shrivelled, dark and leathery appearance.
c	Antemortem burns	• **Line of redness:** Present. • **Redness:** Base of blister is inflamed and swollen; contains protein and chloride; inflammatory reaction is present. • **Vital reaction:** Positive.
d	High voltage burns	• High-tension injuries are either due to direct contact or indirectly by arcing of the flash. • When someone climbs on to an electric pole for suicide or theft of cable, there are chances of arcing when the person comes nearer to the conducting wire. • As much heat is generated in the arcing of the flash and there is knock down by sudden increase of local atmospheric pressure, multiple discrete lesions due to arcing are produced with the blast effect. • These are called **crocodile** burns.

Coming back to the question:

- *Erythema is suggestive of antemortem burns.*

PSM

1. Match the following:

Guidelines	*Studies*
1. CARE	**A. Systematic review and meta-analysis**
2. CONSORT	**B. Randomized controlled trial**
3. PRISMA	**C. Case report**
4. MOOSE	**D. Observational studies**

Lead – Choose the best answer from the codes given below:

A. 1-B, 2-A, 3-D, 4-C
B. 1-C, 2-B, 3-A, 4-D
C. 1-A, 2-B, 3-C, 4-D
D. 1-C, 2-A, 3-B, 4-D

Let's discuss the options:

Option	*Statement*	*Remarks*
1	CARE	• During 2011-2012, a group of clinicians, researchers, and journal editors developed recommendations for the accurate reporting of information in **case reports** that resulted in the CARE (**Ca**se **RE**port) statement and checklist. • They were presented at the 2013 International Congress on Peer Review and Biomedical Publication.
2	CONSORT	• Randomized control trials (**RCTs**) are the gold standard in evaluating and efficiently translating research data into clinical practice. • The CONSORT statement was conceptualized in order to help ascertain standardization and reproducibility of RCTs.

Contd.

		• The CONSORT statement is made up of a 25-item checklist that provides the author with a solid backbone around which to construct and present an RCT. • It sets standard on the trial's design, analysis and interpretation of the results.
3	PRISMA	• The **P**referred **R**eporting **I**tems for **S**ystematic reviews and **M**eta-**A**nalyses (PRISMA) statement, published in 2009, was designed to help systematic reviewers transparently report why the review was done, what the authors did, and what they found. • Over the past decade, advances in systematic review methodology and terminology have necessitated an update to the guideline. • The PRISMA 2020 statement replaces the 2009 statement and includes new reporting guidance that reflects advances in methods to identify, select, appraise and synthesise studies. • The structure and presentation of the items have been modified to facilitate implementation.
4	MOOSE	• MOOSE stands for **M**eta-analysis of **O**bservati**O**nal **S**tudies in **E**pidemiology. • It is a proposed checklist that contains specifications for reporting of meta-analyses of **observational** studies in epidemiology, including background, search strategy, methods, results, discussion and conclusion. • Use of this checklist aims to improve usefulness of meta-analyses for authors, reviewers, editors, readers and decision makers.

Coming back to the question:

Guidelines	*Studies*
1. CARE	*C. Case report*
2. CONSORT	*B. Randomized Controlled Trial*
3. PRISMA	*A. Systematic review and meta-analysis*
4. MOOSE	*D. Observational studies*

2. Statistical method to estimate survival curves when including incomplete observations was given by:

A. Kaplan-Meier
B. Kolmogorov-Smirnov
C. Hall-Wellner
D. Nelson-Aalen

Key points about Kaplan-Meier curve:

- *In 1958, Edward L. Kaplan and Paul Meier collaborated to publish a seminal paper on how to deal with incomplete observations.*
- *Subsequently, the Kaplan Meier curves and estimates of* ***survival*** *data have become a familiar way of dealing with differing survival times (times-to-event), especially when not all the subjects continue in the study.*
- *Examples of when times-to-events may be important end-point variables include cancer survival times, tympanostomy tube duration, onset times of hypocalcemia following parathyroid resection, or duration of nasal congestion following septoplasty.*
- *As illustrated by these examples, 'survival' times need not relate to actual survival with death being the event; the 'event' may be any event of interest.*

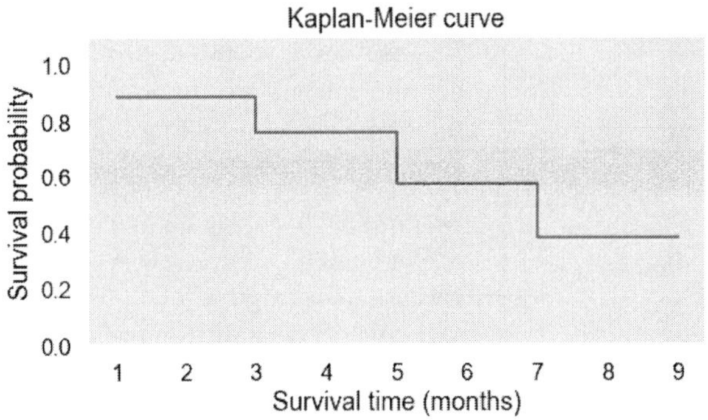

Coming back to the question?

- *Edward L. Kaplan and Paul Meier devised the Statistical method to estimate survival curves when including incomplete observations.*

3. Which of the following disease is transmitted by the vector shown in the image?

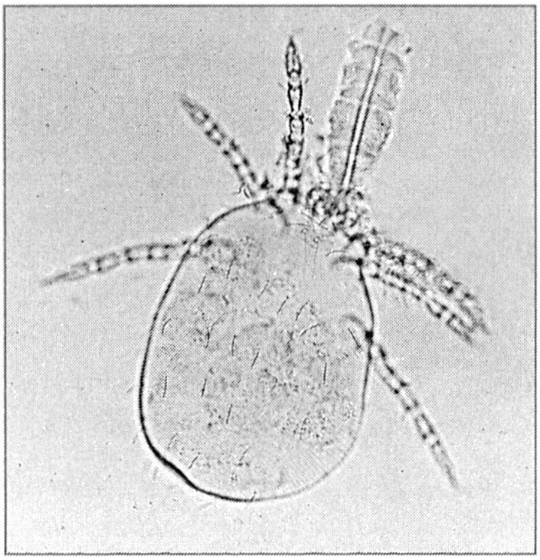

A. Scrub typhus B. KFD
C. Q fever D. Anaplasma

Image shows a trombiculid mite.

Let's discuss the options:

Option	*Statement*	*Remarks*
a	Scrub typhus	• Of the diseases caused by rickettsiae in man, the **most** widespread is scrub typhus. • It exists as a zoonoses in nature between certain species of trombiculid mites and their small mammals (e.g., field mice, rats, shrews). • Scrub typhus is endemic in Northern Japan, South East Asia, the Western Pacific Islands, Eastern Australia, China, Maritime areas and several parts of South-Central Russia, India and Sri Lanka.

Contd.

		• **Causative agent:** Rickettsia tsutsugamushi. • **Reservoir: Trombiculid** mite (Leptotrombidium delinese and L. akamushi). • **Mode of transmission:** By bite of the infected larval mites. • **Incubation period:** Usually 10-12 days; varies from 6 to 21 days. • **Clinical features:** Scrub typhus **resembles** endemic typhus clinically. • The onset is acute with chills and fever, headache, malaise, prostration and a macular rash appearing around the **5th** day of the illness. • Generalized lymphadenopathy and lymphocytosis are common. • One **typical** feature is the punched-out ulcer covered with a blackened scab (eschar), which indicates the location of the mite bite. • The Weil Felix reaction is **strongly** positive with the *Proteus* strain OXK. • **Treatment:** Tetracycline is the drug of **choice**.
b	KFD	• Kyasanur Forest Disease is a febrile disease associated with hemorrhages caused by an arbovirus flavivirus and transmitted to the man by bite of infective ticks. • KFD was **first** recognized in 1957 in Shimoga district of Karnataka state in South India. • Local inhabitants called the disease ‘monkey disease’ because of its association with dead monkeys. • The disease was later named after the locality – Kyasanur Forest – from where the virus was **first** isolated.

Contd.

		• **Causative agent:** Agent KFD virus is a member of group B togaviruses (flaviviruses). • **Reservoir:** Small mammals particularly rats and squirrels are the main reservoir of the virus. • Monkeys are recognized as amplifying hosts for the virus. • Man is an incidental host or dead-end host, and plays **no** role in virus transmission. • **Vector:** The virus has a complex life cycle involving a wide variety of tick-species. • At least 15 species of hard ticks of the genus *Hemaphysalis*, **particularly** *H. spinigera* and *H. turtura* are known to transmit the disease. • KFD has also been isolated from soft ticks. • **Mode of transmission:** Transmission cycle mainly involves monkeys and the ticks. • The disease is transmitted by the bite of infective ticks, especially nymphal stages. • **Incubation period:** 3-8 days. • **Clinical features:** The disease appears with sudden onset of fever, headache and severe myalgia with prostration. • The acute phase lasts for about 2 weeks. • Gastrointestinal disturbances and hemorrhages from nose, gums, stomach and intestine may occur in severe cases. • **Treatment:** Since KFD is a tick-borne disease, control of the ticks should be undertaken by Carbaryl, Fenthion, Naled or Propoxur.

Contd.

c	Q fever	• Q fever is a highly infectious zoonotic disease with worldwide distribution. • It occurs mainly in persons associated with sheep, goats, cattle or other domestic animals. • **Causative agent:** Coxiella burnetti. • **Reservoir:** Cattle, sheep, goats, ticks and some wild animals are natural reservoirs. • **Mode of transmission:** Q fever differs from other rickettsial infections in that there is **no** arthropod involved in transmission to man. • Transmission results from inhalation of infected dust from soil previously contaminated by urine or feces of diseased animals. • **Incubation period:** Usually 2-3 weeks. • **Clinical features:** The disease has an acute onset with fever, chills, general malaise and headache. • The clinical picture is one of influenza or non-bacterial pneumonia **rather** than a typhus fever. • There is **no** rash or local lesion. • **Treatment:** Doxycycline is the drug of **choice**.
d	Anaplas-mosis	• Anaplasmosis is a tickborne disease of ruminants (cattle, sheep, goat etc.). • It is caused by obligate intra-erythrocytic bacteria that infect red blood cells, causing fever and anemia. • Diagnosis relies upon Giemsa-stained blood smears and serologic tests such as ELISA. • **Key** treatments include tetracyclines and imidocarb.

Coming back to the question:

- *Trombiculid mite is the vector for Scrub typhus.*

4. Anthrax bacilli belongs to which category of bioterrorism?

A. Category A
B. Category B
C. Category C
D. All of the above

Let's discuss the options:

Option	*Statement*	*Remarks*
a	Category A	• These agents are the **highest** priority pathogens which pose the **greatest** risk to national security. • These agents can be **easily** disseminated or transmitted from person to person. • Results in **high** mortality and have the potential for **major** public health impact. • Might cause public panic and social disruption. • Require special action for public health preparedness. **Examples:** • **Anthrax** (Bacillus anthracis). • Botulism (Clostridium botulinum toxin). • Plague (Yersinia pestis). • Tularemia (Francisella tularensis). • Smallpox (Variola major).
b	Category B	• These agents are the **second** highest priority pathogens. • They are moderate easy to disseminate. • Result in moderate morbidity rates and **low** mortality rates. • Require specifically enhanced diagnostic capacity.

Contd.

		Examples: • Meliodosis (Burkholderia pseudomallei). • Glanders (Burkholderia mallei). • Brucellosis (Brucella species). • Psittacosis (Chlamydophila psittaci). • Q fever (Coxiella burnetti). • Typhus fever (Rickettsia prowazekii).
c	Category C	• These agents are the third highest priority pathogens. They are emerging pathogens, to which the general population lacks immunity. • These agents **could** be engineered for mass dissemination in the future because of availability, ease of production and ease of dissemination. • They have a potential for high morbidity and mortality rates. **Examples:** • Niaph virus. • Hantavirus. • SARS coronavirus. • Pandemic influenza virus. • MDR-TB. • Yellow fever virus.

Coming back to the question:

- *Bacillus anthracis belongs to Category A of bioterrorism/ bioweapons.*

5. There were 1000 participants in a study which were followed for 25 years. Out of these 1000 participants, 150 developed lung carcinoma. Now these 150 cases were compared with the controls from the same study group. Such type of study is known as:

A. Combined retrospective and prospective cohort study
B. Nested case control study
C. Retrospective cohort study
D. Case control study

Let's discuss the options:

Option	*Statement*	*Remarks*
a	Combined retrospective and prospective cohort study	• In this type of study, both the retrospective and prospective elements are combined. • The cohort is identified from past records, and is assessed of date for the outcome. • The same cohort is followed up prospectively into future for further assessment of outcome.
b	Nested case control study	• In the nested case control study, **cases** of a disease that occur in a defined **cohort** are identified and, for each, a specified number of matched **controls** is selected from among those in the cohort who have not developed the disease by the time of disease occurrence in the case.
c	Retrospective cohort study	• A retrospective cohort study is one in which the outcomes have all occurred before the start of the investigation. • The investigator goes back in time, sometimes 10-30 years, to select his study groups from the existing records of past employment, medical or other records and the traces them forward through time, from a past date fixed on the records, usually up to the present.

Contd.

		• Since a retrospective cohort study depends on past information about the exposure history of the cohort members, it is also known as historical cohort study, prospective study in retrospect and non-concurrent prospective study.
d	Case control study	• A case control study involves two populations – cases and controls. • In case control studies, the unit is the individual rather than the group. • The focus is on a disease or some other health problem that has already developed. • Case control studies are basically comparison studies. • Cases and controls must be comparable with respect to known 'confounding factors' such as age, sex, occupation, social status etc.

Coming back to the question:

- *Nested case control study is a case control study situated within the prospective cohort study.*

6. Which of the following formula is used to calculate standard deviation?

A. $\sqrt{\sum(x-\bar{x})/\eta}$ B. $\sqrt{\sum(x-\bar{x})^2/\eta}$

C. $\sqrt{\sum(x-\bar{x})^3/\eta}$ D. $\sqrt{\sum(x^2-\bar{x}^2)/\eta}$

Key points about Standard deviation:

- *The standard deviation is the **most** frequently used measure of deviation.*

- *In simple terms, it is defined as 'Root – Means – Square – Deviation'.*
- *It is denoted by the Greek letter sigma σ or by the initials S.D.*
- *The standard deviation is calculated from the basic formula:*
    - $\sqrt{\sum(x-\bar{x})^2/\eta}$.
- *When the sample size is more than 30, the above basic formula may be used without modification.*
- *For smaller samples, the above tends to underestimate the standard deviation, and therefore needs correction, which is done by substituting the denominator (η -1) for η.*
- *The modified formula is as follows:*
    - $\sqrt{\sum(x-\bar{x})^2/\eta -1}$.
- *The steps involved in calculating the standard deviation are as follows:*
    - *First of all, take the deviation of each value from the arithmetic mean,* $(x-\bar{x})$.
    - *Then, square each deviation,* $(x-\bar{x})^2$.
    - *Add up the squared deviations,* $\sum(x-\bar{x})^2$.
    - *Divide the result by the number of observations η [or (η -1) in case the sample size is less than 30].*
    - *Then take the square root, which gives the standard deviation.*

Coming back to the question:

- *The formula for calculating standard deviation is* $\sqrt{\sum(x-\bar{x})^2/\eta}$.

7. A child was given DPT vaccine at the age of 10 weeks. After vaccination the child has inconsolable persistent cry. He had fever of more than 40 degrees C. What should be done for next shot?

A. Defer DPT vaccine for next 1 month
B. In next visit (of schedule), give DT in place of DPT
C. Never administer DPT
D. Continue with DPT as per schedule

Key points about DPT vaccine:

- *For immunizing infants, the preparation of* ***choice*** *is DPT.*

- *Firstly, because, the infant can be immunized simultaneously against three diseases, viz., diphtheria, pertussis and tetanus which is a great pain administratively.*
- *Secondly, the pertussis component in DPT vaccine enhances the potency of the diphtheria toxoid.*
- *DPT vaccine should* ***not*** *be frozen. It should be stored in a refrigerator between 2 and 8 degrees C.*
- *Three doses of DPT each of which is usually 0.5 ml, should be considered* ***optimal*** *for primary immunization.*
- *It is associated with higher and more sustained levels of diphtheria and tetanus antitoxin and acceptable level of pertussis reaction, i.e., vaccine efficacy 95 percent.*
- *The current recommendation is to allow an interval of 4 weeks between the 3 doses, with a booster injection at 16-24 months, followed by another booster at the age of 5 to 6 years.*
- *DPT should be administered intramuscular in antero (lateral aspect) of the thigh.*
- *Fever and mild local reactions following DPT immunization are* ***common****.*
- *The* ***most*** *severe complications following DPT immunization are neurological (encephalitis/encephalopathy, prolonged convulsions, infantile spams and Reye's syndrome) and are thought to be due primarily to the pertussis component of the vaccine.*
- *Minor illnesses such as cough, cold, mild fever are* ***not*** *considered contraindications to vaccination, only such children who are seriously ill or need hospitalization are not vaccinated.*
- *DPT should* ***not*** *be repeated if a severe reaction occurred after a previous dose.*
- *Such reactions include collapse or shock-like state,* ***persistent*** *screaming episodes, temperature above* ***40*** *degrees C, convulsions, other neurological symptoms and anaphylactic reactions.*
- *In the case of DPT, subsequent immunization with DT is* ***only*** *recommended, without the pertussis component.*

Coming back to the question:

- *DPT should not be repeated if severe reactions occurred after a previous dose which include persistent screaming episodes and temperature above 40 degrees Celsius. In such cases, subsequent immunization with DT only is recommended.*

8. All of the following are useful in determining normalcy of the data EXCEPT:

A. Mantel-Haenszel statistic
B. Shapiro-Wilk test
C. Histogram
D. Box and Whisker plot

Let's discuss the options:

Option	*Statement*	*Remarks*
a	Mantel Haenszel statistic	• The Mantel-Haenszel statistic (MH) can be used for comparing two cultural groups when the observed item scores are dichotomous (correct-incorrect) and the sum score is used as a proxy for the latent variable. • In a first step, the sum score is reduced to a limited number of score levels. • Within each score level, the odds of correctly versus incorrectly responding are computed within each of the two groups and the ratio of these odds is taken. • Then, the odds ratios are averaged across score levels. • If there is no uniform bias present, the average odds ratio should equal 1. This means that the probability of correctly responding is on average the same in each group for subjects with the same position on the proxy. • If the odds ratio deviates significantly from 1, there is a case for uniform bias. It means that in one cultural group the probability of correctly answering the item is systematically higher than in the other cultural group with the same position on the proxy.

Contd.

		• Because the MH is robust and easy to use, it is one of the most frequently used psychometric methods in item bas research.
b	Shapiro-Wilk test	• The Shapiro-Wilk test can be used to decide whether or not a sample fits a normal distribution, and it is commonly used for small samples. • The Shapiro-Wilk test is essentially a goodness-of-fit test. That is, it examines how close the sample data fit to a normal distribution. • It does this by ordering and standardizing the sample (standardizing refers to converting the data to a distribution with mean μ=0 and standard deviation = 1). • If the sample data perfectly fit a normal distribution, then after this ordering and standardization process the sample would be regularly spaced quantile values of the standard normal distribution. • The Shapiro-Wilk test statistic is basically a measure of how well the ordered and standardized sample quantiles fit the standard normal quantiles.
c	Histogram	• It is a pictorial diagram of frequency distribution. • It consists of a series of block. • The class intervals are given along the horizontal axis and the frequencies along the vertical axis. • The area of each block or rectangle is proportional to the frequency.

Contd.

d	Box and Whisker plot	• The process to abstract a set of data that is estimated using an interval scale is called a box and whisker plot. • It is also called just a box plot. • These are mostly used for data interpretation. • It is one of the types of graphical methods which displays the variation of the data in the dataset. • We can also use the histogram to display the data. But, histogram provides a sufficient display. • Box and Whisker plot is better than histogram as a Box and Whisker diagram will provide additional information as it allows multiple sets of data to be displayed in the same graph.

Coming back to the question:

- *Normalcy of a data can be determined by Shapiro-Wilk test, Histogram and Box and Whisker plot.*

9. Live vaccines are contraindicated in which of the following immunodeficiency disorders?

I. Di George syndrome **II. Ataxia telangiectasia**

III. Wiskott-Aldrich syndrome **IV. Complement deficiency**

Lead – Choose the best answer from the codes given below:

A. I and II B. II and III

C. I, II and IV D. I, II, III and IV

Key points about vaccination in immunodeficiency:

- *Congenital immune deficiencies including* ***complement*** *deficiencies, phagocyte dysfunctions, cell receptor and signal transmission disorders, X-linked agammaglobulinemia which leads to antibody production failure, variable immune deficiencies, severe combined immunodeficiency syndrome, complete* ***Di George*** *syndrome.*

*Wiskott-Aldrich syndrome, adaptive immune deficiencies including **ataxia**-telangiectasia are very important causes of infections, morbidities and mortality.*

- *Inactive vaccines can be **safely** administered in these patients.*
- *Live vaccines should **not** be administered since they may cause severe systemic disease by way of viremia/bacteriemia.*

Coming back to the question:

- *Live vaccines should not be administered in Di George syndrome, Ataxia telangiectasia, Wiskott-Aldrich syndrome and Complement deficiency.*

10. Calculate Kappa coefficient:

	IGRA (Interferon-Gamma Release Assay) suspect TB	***Not TB detected on IGRA (Interferon-Gamma Release Assay)***	***Total***
TST (Tuberculin Skin Test) suspect TB	80	40	**120**
No TB detected on TST (Tuberculin Skin Test)	20	60	**80**
Total	**100**	**100**	**200**

A. 0.5
B. 0.6
C. 0.7
D. 0.4

Key points about Cohen's kappa coefficient:

- *It is a statistic which measures inter-rater agreement for qualitative (categorical) terms.*
- *It is generally thought to be more a robust measure than simple percent agreement calculation, since k takes into account the agreement occurring by chance.*

- *Cohen's kappa measures the agreement between two raters who each classify N items into C mutually exclusive categories.*
- *Formula for calculating kappa coefficient k =* ***p0 − pe/1 − pe***
- *Where:*
    - o ***p0*** *= relative observed agreement among raters.*
    - o ***Pe*** *= the hypothetical probability of chance agreement.*
- *In the given MCQ, there are* ***80*** *cases which are detected as TB by both TST and IGRA and* ***60*** *cases are labelled as no TB by both the tests.*
- *So* ***p0*** *=* ***80 + 60****/200 =* ***0.****7 (200 is total number of cases).*
- *TST detects TB in 120 cases and no TB detected in 80 cases. So TST detected TB in* ***60%*** *cases (120 + 80/200) and does not detect TB in the remaining* ***40%*** *cases.*
- *IGRA detected TB in 100 cases and no TB detected in 100 cases. So IGRA detected TB in* ***50%*** *cases and does not detected TB in remaining* ***50%*** *of cases.*
- *The probability that both of them would be detected TB randomly is* ***0.60*** *×* ***0.50*** *=* ***0.3*** *and the probability that both of them would not detect TB is* ***0.40*** *×* ***0.50*** *=* ***0.2****. Thus, the overall probability of random agreement is* ***pe*** *=* ***0.3*** *+* ***0.2*** *=* ***0.5****.*
- *So now applying formula for calculating kappa coefficient k = p0−pe/1−pe.*
- ***0.****7 -* ***0.5****/1 -* ***0.5*** *=* ***0.****4.*

Coming back to the question:

- *Kappa coefficient from the given data comes out to be 0.4.*

11. All of the following are correct statements related to central tendency EXCEPT:

A. Mode is least affected by extreme value
B. Mean is affected by extreme value
C. Mode is for qualitative data
D. Median look for all observations

Let's discuss the options:

Option	*Statement*	*Remarks*
a, c	Mode	• The mode is the **most** commonly occurring value in a distribution of data. • It is the **most** frequent item or the **most** 'fashionable' value in a series of observations. • The advantages of mode are that it is easy to understand, and is **not** affected by the **extreme** items. • The disadvantages are that the exact location is often uncertain and is often **not** clearly defined. • Therefore, mode is **not** often used in biological or medical statistics.
b	Mean	• The arithmetic mean is **widely** used in statistical calculation. • It is sometimes simply called mean. • To obtain the mean, the individual observations are first added together, and then divided by the number of observations. • The operation of adding together is known as 'summation' and is denoted by the sign $\sum$ or S. • The individual observation is denoted by the sign η and the mean is denoted by the sign $\bar{x}$ (called 'X' bar). • The advantages of the mean are that it is easy to calculate and understand. • The disadvantages are that sometimes it may be unduly influenced by abnormal values in the distribution. • Sometimes it may even look ridiculous; for instance, the average number of children born to a woman in a certain place was found to be 4.76, which nerve occurs in reality. • Mean is **affected** by extreme values.

		• For example, the income of 7 people per day in INR is as follows: 5, 5, 5, 7, 10, 20, 102 (Total = 154). The mean is 154 divided by 7 which is 22. In this example, the income of seventh individual (102 INR) has seriously affected the mean. • Nevertheless, the arithmetic mean is by far the **most** useful of the statistical averages.
d	Median	• The median is an average of a different kind, which does **not** depend upon the total and number of items. • To obtain, the median, the data is arranged in an ascending or descending order of magnitude, and then the value of the **middle** observation is located, which is called the median. • If there are even number of values instead of odd, the median is worked out by taking the average of the two middle values. • Median is **more** nearer the truth, and therefore more representative than the mean. • For example, the income of 7 people per day in INR is as follows: 5, 5, 5, 7, 10, 20, 102. • The median is 7.

Coming back to the question:

- *Median looks for middle observation (and not for all the observations).*

ENT

1. Arrange the following structure as per origin of BERA waves:

I. Lateral lemniscus
II. Auditory nerve
III. Superior olivary complex
IV. Cochlear nuclei
V. Inferior colliculus

Lead – Choose the best answer from the codes given below:

A. I → II → III → V → IV
B. II → III → V → I → IV
C. II → IV → III → I → V
D. I → IV → III → II → V

Key points about Brainstem Evoked Response Audiometry/BERA/ Auditory Brainstem Response/ABR/Auditory Nerve and Brainstem Evoked Potentials/ABEP:

- *Like OAEs (OtoAcoustic Emissions), BERA is an objective test.*
- *But unlike OAEs which measure the spontaneous electrical activity from the cochlea (outer hair cells of the Organ of Corti), BERA tests the electrical activity occurring in the auditory pathway (situated in the brainstem that is why the name) within 10 milli-second in response to a sound stimulus.*
- *BERA finds the integrity of central auditory pathways, which consists of 8th nerve, pons, midbrain and forebrain.*
- *In a normal person, 5-7 electrical waves are recorded in the form of a graph with latency (i.e., time in milli-second taken for the wave to appear after the stimulus sound is given) on the x-axis and amplitude on the y-axis.*
- *These waves come from the different areas of the auditory pathway.*
- *The wave V is the most prominent and easily identifiable and hence, the most important wave of BERA.*
- *Wave I originates from* ***E****ighth CN/Auditory Nerve.*
- *Wave II originates from* ***C****ochlear nucleus (pons).*
- *Wave III originates from Superior* ***O****livary complex (pons).*
- *Wave IV originates from* ***L****ateral lemniscus (pons).*

- *Wave V originates from **I**nferior colliculus (midbrain).*

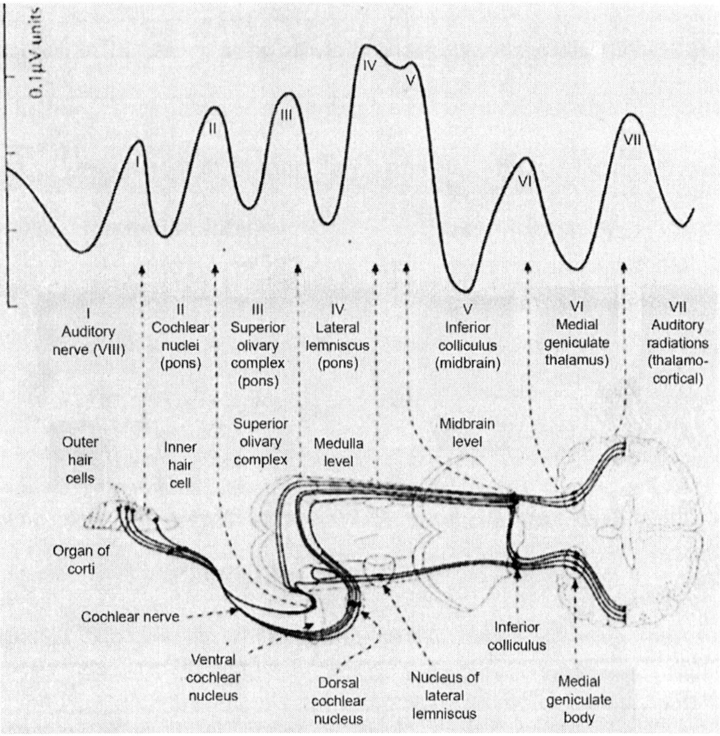

Coming back to the question:

- *Sequence of anatomical structures giving rise to BERA waves is Auditory nerve → Cochlear nucleus → Superior Olivary complex → Lateral lemniscus → Inferior colliculus.*

2. The nerve block performed in the image shown below is:

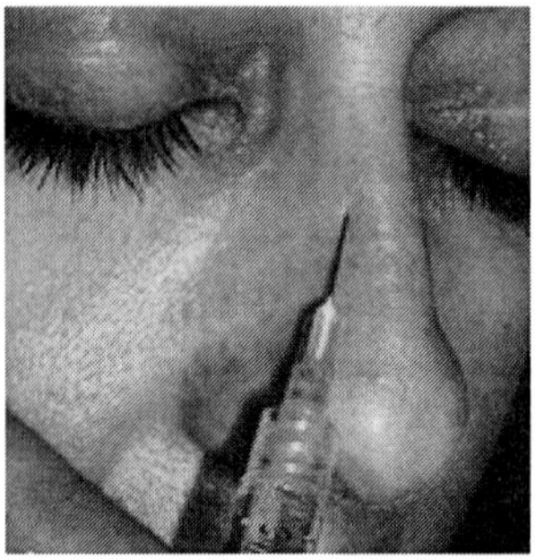

A. Sphenopalatine nerve block
B. Anterior ethmoidal nerve block
C. Nasociliary nerve block
D. Infraorbital nerve block

Key points about anterior ethmoidal nerve:

- *The anterior ethmoidal nerve is a terminal branch of the nasociliary nerve (a branch of ophthalmic division (CN V_1) of trigeminal nerve).*
- *It branches near the medial wall of the orbit.*
- *The anterior ethmoidal nerve arises only after the nasociliary has given off its four branches (the ramus communicans to the ciliary ganglion, the long ciliary nerves, the infratrochlear nerve, and the posterior ethmoidal nerve).*
- *Anterosuperior part of the nasal cavity (lateral wall and septum) is supplied by anterior ethmoidal nerve.*

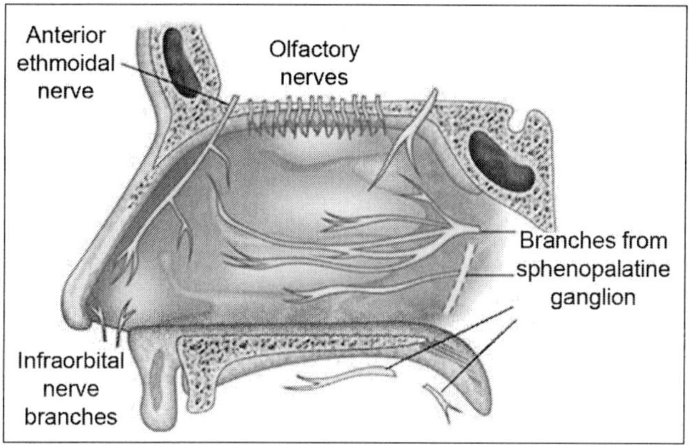

Coming back to the question:

- *The nerve block performed in the given image is anterior ethmoidal nerve block.*

3. Arrange the following structures as per their sequence in auditory pathway:

I. Lateral lemniscus **II. Eighth cranial nerve**
III. Superior olivary nucleus **IV. Medial geniculate body**
V. Inferior nucleus **VI. Cochlear nucleus**
VII. Auditory cortex

Lead – Choose the best answer from the codes given below:

A. I → II → III → IV → V → VI → VII
B. II → III → V → VII → I → VI → IV
C. II → VI → III → I → V → IV → VII
D. IV → I → VII → VI → III → II → V

Key points about auditory neural pathway:

- *The auditory pathway from peripheral to center consists of* ***ECOLIMA****.*
- ***E****ighth nerve.*
- ***C****ochlear nuclei.*
- ***O****livary complex (superior).*
- ***L****ateral lemniscus.*
- ***I****nferior colliculus.*
- ***M****edial geniculate body.*
- ***A****uditory cortex.*

Coming back to the question:

- *Sequence of Auditory pathway: Eighth nerve → Cochlear nucleus → Superior Olivary complex → Lateral lemniscus → Inferior colliculus → Medial geniculate body → Auditory cortex.*

OPHTHALMOLOGY

1. Which of the following is true regarding glaucoma?

A. Visual field defect is not associated with optic nerve head changes
B. Kinetic perimetry is the best diagnostic modality for monitoring field changes in glaucoma
C. In static perimetry, the stimulus is moving but with fixed luminance
D. Earliest change is isopter contraction and baring of blind spot

Let's discuss the options:

Option	*Statement*	*Remarks*
a	Visual field defect is not associated with optic nerve head changes	• False statement. • Visual field defects appear only after about 40% of axons have been damaged and subsequently the field defects usually run parallel to the changes at the optic nerve head and continue to progress is intraocular pressure/IOP is not controlled.
b	Kinetic perimetry is the best diagnostic modality for monitoring field changes in glaucoma	• False statement. • In kinetic perimetry, the stimulus of known luminance is moved from a peripheral non-seeing pint towards the centre till it is perceived to establish the isopters. • Various methods of kinetic perimetry are: Confrontation method, Lister's perimetry, tangent screen scotometry and Goldmann's perimetry. • Lister's perimeter is **not** in much use now-a-days, though it is useful for peripheral field charting.

Contd.

		• Goldmann perimeter is **not** in much use presently. • Most of the kinetic methods of field testing are done manually. • Presently, automated perimetry (static perimetry) has almost completely **replaced** the manual perimetry.
c	In static perimetry, the stimulus is moving but with fixed luminance	• False statement. • Static perimetry involves presenting a stimulus at a **predetermined** position for a present duration with **varying** luminance in the field of vision. • Various methods of static perimetry adopted are Goldmann perimetry, Friedmann perimetry, automated perimetry.
d	Earliest change is isopter contraction and baring of blind spot	• True statement. • Isopter contraction refers to mild generalized constriction of central as well as peripheral field. • It is the **earliest** visual field defect occurring in glaucoma. • However, it is of limited diagnostic value, as it may also occur in many other conditions. • Baring of the blind spot is also considered to be an **early** glaucomatous change, but is very nonspecific and thus of limited diagnostic value. • Baring of the blind spot means exclusion of the blind spot from the central field due to inward curve of the outer boundary of 30^0 central field.

Coming back to the question:

- *Earliest change in glaucoma include isopter contraction and baring of blind spot.*

2. How many order neurons are involved in vestibulo-ocular reflex?

A. 1 B. 2
C. 3 D. 4

Key points about VOR/Vestibulo-ocular reflex:

- *VOR acts by activating eye muscles to create eye movement in the exact speed but in opposite direction of head movement so as to stabilize retinal images.*
- *Vestibular information comes into the brainstem via the cranial nerve VIII.*
- *Signal enter the vestibular nuclear complex/VNC, located in the medulla and pons.*
- *Using **first**-order sensory neurons of the cranial nerve VIII, most of the semicircular canal inputs synapse at the superior and medial nuclei of VNC.*
- *The medial longitudinal fasciculus is used to send **second**-order sensory neuron signals ipsi- and contralaterally to cranial nerves III, IV and VI.*
- *Lastly, a **third**-order motor neuron is responsible for stimulating the extraocular muscles that cause the conjugate eye movements.*
- *VOR involves three parts:*
  - o *A peripheral sensory apparatus [which consists of a set of motion sensors: the semicircular canals and the otolith organs (saccule and utricle)].*
  - o *A central processing mechanism.*
  - o *A motor output (which are the eye muscles).*
- *Application of VOR in clinical practice includes Oculocephalic reflex/Doll's eye reflex, which examines **three** cranial nerves*

(oculomotor, abducens and vestibulocochlear nerve), brainstem nuclei and overall brainstem functions.

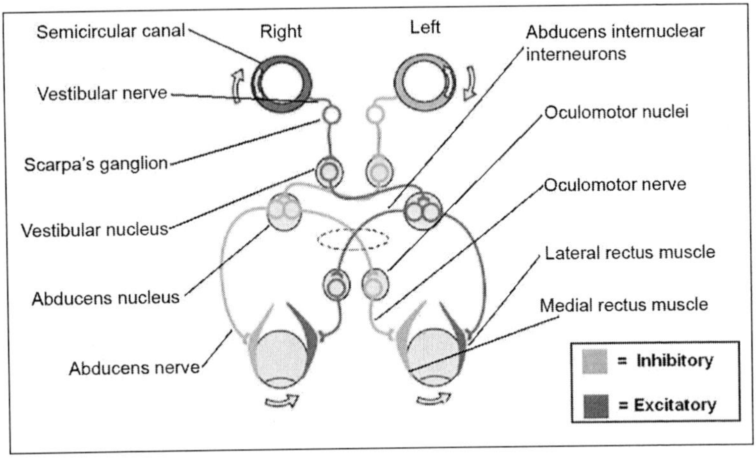

Coming back to the question:

- *Three order neurons are involved in vestibulo-ocular reflex.*

3. Which of the following are examples of Direct Goniolenses?

I. Richardon-Shaffer	**II. Zeiss**
III. Goldmann	**IV. Koeppe**

Lead – Choose the best answer from the codes given below:

A. I and II	B. II and III
C. I, II and III	D. I and IV

Key points about Gonioscopy:

- *Owing to the lack of transparency of corneoscleral junction and total internal reflection of light (emitted from angle structures) at anterior surface of cornea, it is not possible to visualize the angle of anterior chamber directly.*
- *Therefore, a device (goniolens) is used to divert the beam of light and this technique of biomicroscopic examination of the angle of anterior chamber is called gonioscopy.*

- *Types of goniolens:*
    - o *Indirect: They provide a mirror image of the opposite angle.*
    - o *Direct: They provide a direct view of the angle.*
- *Angle structures seen from behind forward are:*
    - o *Root of the iris.*
    - o *Anteromedial surface of the ciliary body (ciliary band).*
    - o *Scleral spur.*
    - o *Trabecular meshwork and Schlemm's canal.*
    - o *Schwalbe's line.*
- *Applications of gonioscopy:*
    - o *Classification of glaucoma into open angle and closed angle based on configuration of the angle.*
    - o *Localization of foreign bodies, abnormal blood vessels or tumours in the angle.*
    - o *Demonstration of extent of peripheral anterior synechiae (PAS) and hence planning of glaucoma surgery.*
    - o *Direct goniolens is used for goniotomy.*

Let's discuss the options:

Option	*Statement*	*Remarks*
I	Richardson-Shaffer	• Direct goniolens
II	Zeiss	• Indirect goniolens
III	Goldmann	• Indirect goniolens
IV	Koeppe	• Direct goniolens

Coming back to the question:

- *Richardson-Shaffer and Koeppe goniolens are examples of direct goniolenses.*

4. Identify the structure marked with black arrow in the image given below:

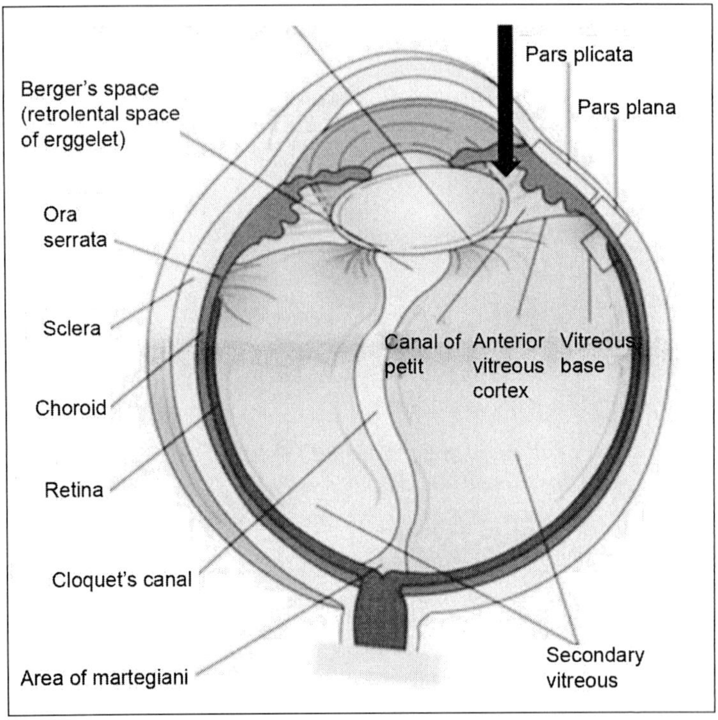

A. Weigert's ligament
B. Hyaloid canal
C. Canal of Hannover
D. Canal of Petit

Key points about arrangement of zonular fibres of lens:

- *According to new concept the zonular fibres run a more or less complex but continuous course from ora serrata to the edge of lens.*
- *However, for purpose of description only, the zonular complex can be divided into the following parts.*
- ***Pars orbicularis**: It refers to the feltwork of zonular fibres which line pars plana part of the ciliary body.*
- ***Zonular plexuses**: It refers to the intervening network of zonular fibres which are attached between ciliary processes in the region of the pars plicata part of ciliary body.*
- ***Zonular fork:** It refers to the consolidated bundle of zonular fibres which bend at right angle from the anterior margin of pars plicata towards the lens after dividing into three zonular limbs:*

- o *Anterior zonular limb: These fibres are denser and insert on the anterior lens capsule about 1.5 mm from the equator.*
- o *Equatorial zonular limb: These fibres are sparse and fan out in a brush-like manner to get inserted into the lens capsule of equatorial region.*
- o *Posterior zonular limb: These fibres are inserted on the posterior lens capsule about 1.25 mm from the equator.*

Let's discuss the options:

Option	*Statement*	*Remarks*
a	Weigert's ligament	• Weigert's ligament is a circular zone of adhesion, 8-9 mm in diameter, between the gel and the posterior lens capsule. • It is the junction between the anterior hyaloid membrane and the expanded anterior portion of the Cloquet's canal.
b	Hyaloid canal	• Hyaloid canal/Cloquet's canal/ Stilling's canal is a small transparent canal running through the vitreous body from the optic nerve disc (at the punctum caecum) to the lens. • It is formed by an invagination of the hyaloid membrane, which encloses the vitreous body.
c	Canal of Hannover	• The space between pre-equatorial (anterior) and post-equatorial (posterior) zonules is called Canal of Hannover. • It is filled with the fine fibres of the equatorial zonules.
d	Canal of Petit	• The space between the post-equatorial (posterior) zonules and hyaloid zonules is known as canal of Petit.

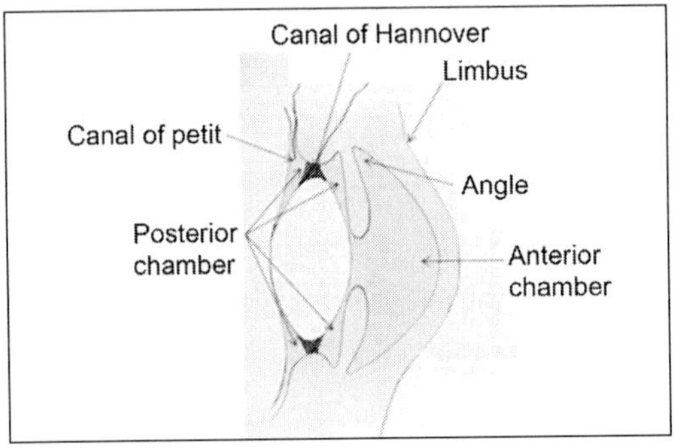

Coming back to the question:

- *The space between pre-equatorial (anterior) and post-equatorial (posterior) zonules is called Canal of Hannover.*

5. Images are shown below, from a patient, before and after topical application of Phenylephrine. Most likely diagnosis:

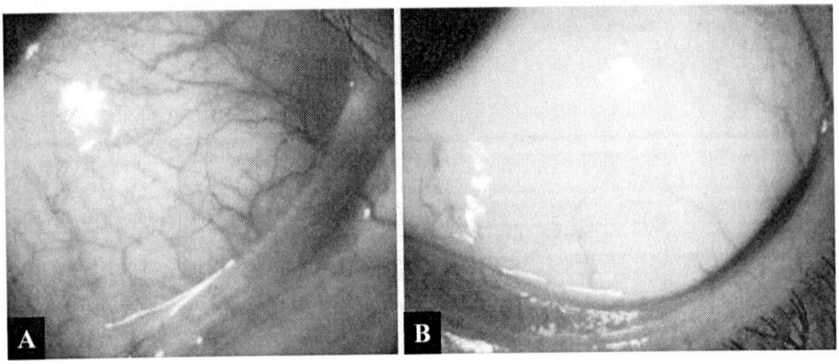

A. Acute bacterial conjunctivitis
B. Phlyctenular conjunctivitis
C. Nodular episcleritis
D. Nodular non-necrotizing scleritis

Key points about Episcleritis:

- *Episcleritis is an inflammatory disorder involving the episcleral tissue that lies superficial to the sclera, just beneath Tenon's capsule.*
- *It is seen more frequently in young to middle-aged women.*
- *Episcleritis is usually mild, characterized by slight conjunctival injection and the presence of foreign body sensation.*
- *The episode often resolves without treatment, but can recur.*

- *Inflamed episcleral blood vessels tend to have a salmon color in natural light, radiate from the limbus, and can be moved over the sclera with a cotton-tipped applicator.*
- *In addition, these more superficial vessels will blanch after administration of topical* ***Phenylepinephrine****.*

Let's discuss the options:

Option	*Statement*	*Remarks*
a	Acute bacterial conjunctivitis	• Acute bacterial conjunctivitis is characterized by marked conjunctival hyperaemia and mucopurulent discharge from the eye. • So, clinically it is called acute mucopurulent conjunctivitis. • It is **most** common type of bacterial conjunctivitis.
b	Phlyctenular conjunctivitis	• Presence of one or more whitish raised nodules on the bulbar conjunctiva near the limbus, with hyperaemia usually of the surrounding conjunctiva, in a child living in bad hygienic conditions (most of the times) are the **diagnostic** features of the Phlyctenular conjunctivitis.
c	Nodular episcleritis	• It is characterized by a pink or purple flat nodule surrounded by injection, usually situated 2-3 mm away from the limbus. • The nodule is firm, tender, can be **moved** separately from the sclera and the overlying conjunctiva also moves freely.
d	Nodular non-necrotizing scleritis	• Non-necrotizing anterior nodular scleritis is characterized by one or two hard, purplish elevated **immovable** scleral nodules, usually situated near the limbus.

Coming back to the question:

- *More superficial vessels in nodular episcleritis will blanch after administration of topical Phenylepinephrine.*

6. Arrange the following in decreasing order of preference for staining a dry eye:

I. Lissamine green **II. Rose Bengal**

III. Fluorescein dye

Lead – Choose the best answer from the codes given below:

A. I → II → III B. III → II → I

C. II → III → I D. III → I → II

Key points about staining for dry eye:

- *The ocular surface is **most** commonly stained with fluorescein dye.*
- *The fluorescein is applied on a moistened sterile strip of paper to the inner lining of the lower eyelid or applied in an eye drop mixed with a topical anaesthetic.*
- *The ophthalmic strips might be mildly irritating and the drop may briefly burn.*
- *When abnormal or missing epithelial cells are stained with fluorescein and observed under the cobalt blue light, they appear bright green.*
- *Bright green areas of the cornea may indicate dry eye, as well as other conditions.*
- *Other less commonly utilized stains are Lissamine green and Rose Bengal.*
- *Lissamine green and Rose Bengal have similar staining characteristics for evaluating the conjunctiva.*
- *Lissamine green is **less** toxic and **better** tolerated than Rose Bengal.*

Coming back to the question:

- *The preferred stain for dry eye is Fluorescein dye followed by Lissamine green and least preferred is Rose Bengal stain.*

MEDICINE

1. A mother while kissing the child, finds the sweat of the child to be salty. Which of the following channel is affected?

A. Sodium channel
B. Potassium channel
C. Chloride channel
D. Iodide channel

Clinical presentation is indicative of cystic fibrosis.

Key points about Cystic fibrosis/CF:

- *CF is the **most** common, autosomal recessive disorder, with the basic defect in the gene located on the long arm of chromosome 7, which results in the deficiency of cystic fibrosis transmembrane conductance regulatory protein (CFTCR).*
- *CFTCR is a chloride channel activator, activated by a combination of phosphorylation of protein kinase A and binding of ATP.*
- *This genetic defect results in reduction in the movement of in and out of the cell and a reduction in the amount of water in the secretions.*
- *Failure of the **chloride** channel to reabsorb chloride leads to loss of sodium onto the skin surface and a subsequent fluid loss. This causes the **pathognomonic** salty skin seen with CF.*
- *CF is a multisystem disease involving lung, pancreas, sweat glands and urogenital tract.*
- *Respiratory/Cardiovascular:*
    - o *Bronchiectasis.*
    - o *Sinusitis.*
    - o *Cor pulmonale.*
- *Intestinal:*
    - o *Meconium ileus.*
    - o *Volvulus.*
- *Pancreatic:*
    - o *Nutritional deficit and growth failure due to pancreatic insufficiency.*
    - o *Steatorrhoea.*

   - *Diabetes mellitus.*
- *Hepatobiliary:*
   - *Atrophic gallbladder.*
   - *Focal biliary cirrhosis.*
   - *Portal hypertension.*
- *Male reproductive system:*
   - *Sterility (absent or defective vas deferens).*
- *Female reproductive system:*
   - *Decreased fertility (increased viscosity of vaginal secretions).*

Coming back to the question:

- *Sweat of the child is salty in cystic fibrosis, which is because of affection of chloride channels.*

2. A lady presented to the OPD with the complaints of skin thickening. She also had history of numbness in fingers on exposure to cold. She finds difficulty in walking and climbing stairs. Her investigations were: ANA – positive, CPK – elevated and Muscle biopsy showed perivascular inflammatory cell infiltration. Which of the following is the most specific antibody for this disorder?

A. Anti-U_3 RNP
B. Anti-PM/SCL
C. Anti-topoisomerase-1
D. Anti-centromere

Clinical presentation is indicative of systemic sclerosis with polymyositis (Systemic sclerosis Overlap syndrome).

Key points about Systemic Sclerosis Overlap syndrome:

- *SSc/Systemic sclerosis is a heterogeneous, multisystem, chronic disorder, leading to **fibrosis** of the skin and many internal organs.*
- *Severe **Raynaud's** phenomenon is usually the presenting complaint and may precede other features of the disease by months or years.*
- *Antinuclear-antibodies/**ANA** are seen in about 50% of patients of SSc.*
- *Symptoms of SSc occur in combination with those of other connective tissue diseases/CTD, described as SSc-overlap syndrome.*
- *SSc-overlap syndrome is generally considered when musculoskeletal involvement (**myositis**, arthritis) or clinical signs of other rheumatic diseases are substantially greater than usually found in SSc patients.*

- *Musculoskeletal involvement, including joints, tendons and muscles, is the **most** frequent clinical feature, highlighting the difference to other SSc forms.*
- *Investigations in Polymyositis:*
    - o *Serum enzymes (**CPK**, aldolase, AST, LDH and ALT) are increased.*
    - o *Muscle biopsy reveals inflammatory cell infiltrates, destruction of muscle fibres with a phagocytic reaction, and **perivascular** (or perineural) inflammatory cell infiltration (**hallmark** of polymyositis).*

Let's discuss the options:

Option	*Statement*	*Remarks*
a	Anti-U_3 RNP	• Associated with diffuse and limited cutaneous SSc, skeletal myopathy and pulmonary hypertension.
b	Anti-PM/SCL	• Associated with overlap (SSc, Polymyositis).
c	Anti-topoisomerase-1	• Associated with diffuse cutaneous SSc.
d	Anti-centromere	• Associated with limited cutaneous SSc.

Coming back to the question:

- *Autoantibody associated with Systemic Sclerosis Overlap syndrome is anti-PM/SCL.*

3. Match the following:

Feature	*Condition*
1. Trisomy 13	**A. Huntington disease**
2. Trisomy 18	**B. Edward syndrome**
3. Trinucleotide repeated sequence	**C. Patau syndrome**
4. Hemoglobin point mutation of Glutamine to Valine	**D. Sickle cell anemia**

Lead – Choose the best answer from the codes given below:

A. 1-B, 2-A, 3-D, 4-C
B. 1-C, 2-B, 3-A, 4-D
C. 1-A, 2-B, 3-C, 4-D
D. 1-C, 2-A, 3-B, 4-D

Let's discuss the options:

Option	*Statement*	*Remarks*
1	Trisomy 13	• It is also known as **Patau** syndrome. • Polydactyly, flexion deformity of fingers, simian crease, microcephaly, holoprosencephaly, cleft lip and palate and low set malformed ears.
2	Trisomy 18	• It is also known as **Edward** syndrome. • Prominent occiput, low set malformed ears and micrognathia together with clenched fists and rocker bottom feet.
3	Trinucleotide repeated sequence	• CAG nucleotide repeat sequence is a feature of **Huntington's** disease/HD. • Huntington disease is an autosomal dominant disease, characterised by movement disorders and dementia. • Diagnostic triad: Dementia, emotional disturbance and autosomal dominance (familial). • There is profound loss of striatal neurons occurs in the caudate nucleus. • Gene for HD is located on chromosome 4p and encodes protein Huntingtin. • Normal Huntingtin gene contains 6 to 35 copies of CAG repeat. • Trinucleotide repeat is a characteristic feature, resulting in Huntingtin protein aggregation in neurons and as intranuclear inclusions.

Contd.

4	Hemoglobin point mutation of Glutamine to Valine	• **Sickle** cell anemia is a hemolytic anemia resulting from the homozygous inheritance of a gene which causes an amino acid substitution in the hemoglobin molecule (beta-6 glutamate → valine) creating HbS due to point mutation. • HbS shows polymerization, when hemoglobin is deoxygenated, which in turn results in hemolytic anemia, micro-vascular obstruction and ischemic tissue damage. • RBCs with HbS acquires a sickle or holly-leaf shape. • HbS confers protection against falci-parum malaria. • It is common in black Africans and their worldwide descendants.

Coming back to the question:

Feature	***Condition***
1. Trisomy 13	*C. Patau syndrome*
2. Trisomy 18	*B. Edward syndrome*
3. Trinucleotide repeated sequence	*A. Huntington disease*
4. Hemoglobin point mutation of Glutamine to Valine	*D. Sickle cell anemia*

4. All of the following are examples of high cardiac output heart failure states EXCEPT:

A. Anemia
B. Systemic arteriovenous fistula
C. Cor pulmonale
D. Beri-Beri

Key points about High cardiac output heart failure:

- *The normal heart fails to maintain a normal or increased output, in the face of grossly elevated requirements.*

- *Here the cardiac output is above the normal range, but it falls from the original levels as heart failure sets in.*
- *Features of right ventricular failure predominate at first, but later left ventricular failure becomes evident.*
- *It is difficult to determine if the patient with high output states has developed cardiac failure.*
- *The only clue to the development of CCF in these patients may be the presence of shortened circulatory time.*
- *Examples:*
    - o *Thyrotoxicosis.*
    - o *Anemia.*
    - o *Beri-beri.*
    - o *Arteriovenous fistula.*
    - o *Pregnancy.*

Coming back to the question:

- *Cor pulmonale does not come under high cardiac output state.*

5. Which of the following is a true statement regarding transfusion products?

A. Cryoprecipitate is stored at 20-24 degrees C
B. Fresh Frozen Plasma can be stored at -30 degrees C for 2 years
C. Platelets can be stored at 20-24 degrees C for 5 days
D. Packed RBCs can be stored at -15 degrees C with SAGM for 3 weeks

Let's discuss the options:

Option	*Statement*	*Remarks*
a	Cryoprecipitate is stored at 20-24 degrees C	• False statement. • Cryoprecipitate is stored at -20º to -40º C and the shelf life is 12 months.
b	Fresh Frozen Plasma can be stored at -30 degrees C for 2 years	• False statement. • FFP is stored at -20º to -40º C and the shelf life is 12 months.

Contd.

c	Platelets can be stored at 20-24 degrees C for 5 days	• True statement. • Platelet concentrates are stored at room temperature (20^0 to 24^0 C) with agitation and the shelf life is 5 days.
d	Packed RBCs can be stored at -15 degrees C with SAGM for 3 weeks	• False statement. • Red cells are stored at 2 to 6^0 C with a shelf life of 35 days. • Additive solution containing combinations of Saline, Adenine, Glucose and Mannitol (SAGM) provides extended shelf life of RBC up to 42 days with increased functional viability.

Coming back to the question:

- *Platelet concentrates are stored at room temperature (with agitation) and the shelf life is 5 days.*

6. All of the following are related to massive blood transfusion EXCEPT:

A. Hypothermia B. Hypokalemia
C. Hypocalcemia D. Metabolic alkalosis

Key points about Massive blood transfusion:

- *Blood transfusion of more than 5L over a period of 24 hours is termed as massive blood transfusion.*
- *It is required in:*
  - o *Gunshot injury with hemodynamic compromise.*
  - o *Coronary artery bypass graft surgery.*
  - o *Ruptured aneurysm of abdominal aorta.*
- *Current protocol is:*
  - o *6 units of packed RBC.*
  - o *6 units of fresh frozen plasma.*
  - o *6 units of platelets.*
  - o *The recommended ratio of blood components is 1:1:1.*

Let's discuss the options:

Option	*Statement*	*Remarks*
a	Hypothermia	• True statement. • Fast infusion of the blood (at 4° C) can cause **hypothermia** resulting in sluggish circulation.
b	Hypokalemia	• False statement. • Post-expiry date blood transfusion results in hemolysis resulting in **hyperkalemia**. • This can trigger ventricular fibrillation.
c	Hypocalcemia	• True statement. • Citrate ion binds with ionized calcium ion resulting in decreased availability of calcium (**hypocalcemia**) resulting in tetany. • Death in tetany usually occurs due to laryngospasm.
d	Metabolic alkalosis	• True statement. • Citrate toxicity leads to elevated bicarbonate levels in the body and metabolic **alkalosis**.

Coming back to the question:

- *Post-expiry date blood transfusion results in hemolysis resulting in hyperkalemia.*

7. Arrange the following in order of location on left chest wall, going superior to inferior:

I. Tricuspid **II. Pulmonary**

III. Mitral **IV. Aortic**

Lead – Choose the best answer from the codes given below:

A. II → III → IV B. IV → III → I

C. II → I → III D. III → I → II

Let's discuss the auscultation areas:

No.	*Area*	*Remarks*
1	Aortic	• It is over the **right** 2nd intercostal space, close to the sternum. • On this area, the sound produced by the closure of aortic valve (second heart sound) is heard well.
2	Pulmonary	• Pulmonary area is on the left 2nd intercostal space, close to the sternum. • Sound produced by the closure of pulmonary valve (second heart sound) is heard well in this area.
3	Tricuspid	• Tricuspid area corresponds to the lower left parasternal area. • Sound produced by the closure of tricuspid valve (first heart sound) is transmitted well into this area.
4	Mitral	• Mitral area is in the left 5th intercostal space, about 10 inch away from the midline (midclavicular line). • Sound produced by the closure of mitral valve (first heart sound) is transmitted well into this area. • It is also called **apex** beat area because apex beat is felt in this area.

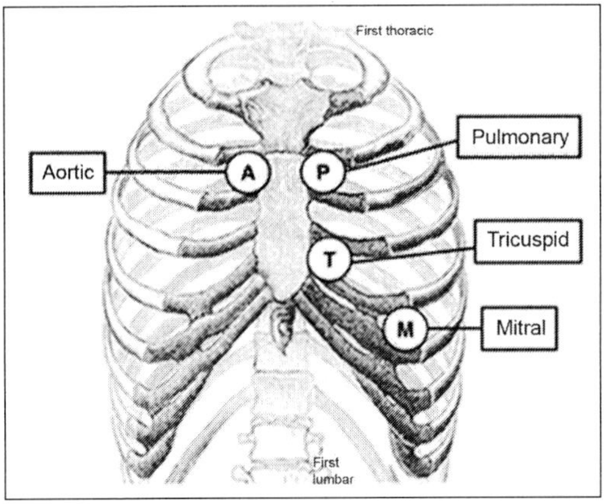

Coming back to the question:

- *Going above downwards, auscultatory areas on the left side of chest wall are pulmonary, tricuspid and mitral.*

8. Which of the following does NOT come in definition of severe COVID illness?

A. PaO_2/FiO_2 of 200 mm Hg
B. Lung infiltrates involving 42% of lung area
C. SpO_2 of 87% on room air
D. Respiratory rate of 32/minute

Let's discuss the options:

Option	*Statement*	*Remarks*
a	PaO_2/FiO_2 of 200 mm Hg	• True statement. • Individuals who have a ratio of arterial partial pressure of oxygen to fraction of inspired oxygen (PaO_2/FiO_2) **<300 mm Hg** are categorized as severe COVID illness.
b	Lung infiltrates involving 42% of lung area	• False statement. • Individuals who have lung infiltrates **>50%** are categorized as severe COVID illness.
c	SpO_2 of 87% on room air	• True statement. • Individuals who have a SpO_2 of **<94%** on room air at sea level are categorized as severe COVID illness.
d	Respiratory rate of 32/minute	• True statement. • Individuals who have a respiratory rate of **>30** breaths/minute are categorized as severe COVID illness.

Coming back to the question:

- *Individuals who have lung infiltrates >50% are categorized as severe COVID illness.*

9. Which of the following are true statements regarding kidney biopsy?

I. If the patient is passing large clots in urine after kidney biopsy, think of hematoma

II. After kidney biopsy, observe the patient for at least 24 hours

III. Kidney should be biopsied in a suspected case of systemic amyloidosis with renal involvement

IV. Focal segmental glomerulosclerosis cannot be diagnosed on percutaneous biopsy

Lead – Choose the best answer from the codes given below:

A. I and II
B. II and III
C. I, II and III
D. I, II and IV

Let's discuss the options:

Option	*Statement*	*Remarks*
I	If the patient is passing large clots in urine after kidney biopsy, think of hematoma	• True statement. • Perinephric **hematoma** is one of the complications that can occur post renal biopsy. • Small hematomas are common, but large hematomas are uncommon.
II	After kidney biopsy, observe the patient for at least 24 hours	• True statement. • Based on the recognition of most complications within 24 hours, in-hospital observation of **24** hours is considered optimal.
III	Kidney should be biopsied in a suspected case of systemic amyloidosis with renal involvement	• False statement. • Histological diagnosis of amyloidosis can be done by **abdominal** fat biopsy or rectal biopsy.

Contd.

IV	Focal segmental glomerulosclerosis cannot be diagnosed on percutaneous biopsy	• False statement. • Focal Segmental Glomerulosclerosis accounts for 30% of nephrotic syndrome in adults and 50% of all steroid resistant cases. • In 'classic FSGS', sclerosis is focal involving <50% of the glomeruli and segmental involving <50% of the glomerular tuft. • The remaining part of the glomerular tuft and the other glomeruli are normal. • Two important **clues** in the biopsy favour the diagnosis. They are abnormally enlarged glomeruli, presence of interstitial fibrosis and tubular atrophy. • Under electron microscopy, there is foot process effacement in sclerotic and non-sclerotic glomeruli.

Coming back to the question:

- *After kidney biopsy, if the patient is passing large clots in urine, think of hematoma and observe the patient for at least 24 hours.*

10. A 65 years old male is being treated for severe breathlessness. There is no significant past medical history. He is having fever with a total leucocyte count of 19,000. His respiratory rate is 33 breaths/minute. His serum creatinine is 1.45 mg/dL and BUN of 45. Sputum shows 2+ pus cells and 1+ epithelial cells. His SpO_2 is 87% on 6L oxygen with nasal cannula. Chest X-ray is shown below. He is confused. Rhinovirus is demonstrated in anterior nares. The patient is shifted to ICU. What should be given to such a patient?

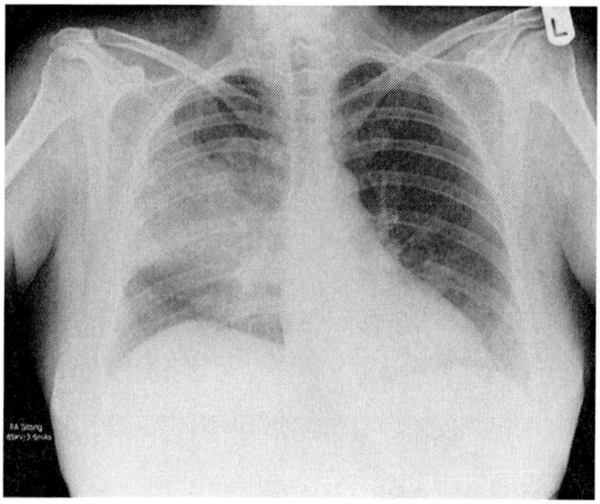

A. Azithromycin alone
B. Piperacillin/Tazobactam + Ciprofloxacin
C. Amoxycillin + Clavulanic acid
D. Ceftazidime + Azithromycin

Clinical presentation and chest X-ray are indicative of severe community acquired pneumonia.

Key points about Community acquired pneumonia:

- *Assessment is done by CURB 65.*
- ***C**onfusion.*
- ***U**rea >7 mmol/L.*
- ***R**espiratory rate >30/minute.*
- ***B**P: Systolic <90, Diastolic <60 mm of Hg.*
- *Age >**65** years.*
- *Score:*
    - o *0: Out-patient.*
    - o *2: In-patient.*
    - o *3: Intensive care unit.*
- *Treatment guidelines:*
    - o *Out-patients: Clarithromycin/Azithromycin/Doxycycline.*
    - o *In-patients (non-ICU):*
        - ♦ *Moxifloxacin/Gemifloxacin/Levofloxacin.*

- ♦ *Beta-lactam Ceftriaxone/Cefotaxime/Ertapenem + Macrolide.*
- ♦ *Clarithromycin/Azithromycin.*

o *In-patients **(ICU)**: Beta-lactam Ceftriaxone/Cefotaxime/ Ampicilin-Sulbactam + Azithromycin/Fluoroquinolones.*

Coming back to the question:

- *A case of severe community acquired pneumonia, who is admitted in ICU should be managed by Ceftazidime + Azithromycin.*

11. What is the mechanism of action of plasmapheresis in thrombotic thrombocytopenic purpura?

A. Destroys ADAMTS 13 protein

B. Inhibits the enzyme which forms ADAMTS 13 protein

C. Promotes formation of ADAMTS 13 antibodies

D. Removes anti-ADAMTS13 antibodies

Key points about TTP:

- *It is a multisystem disease characterized by thrombocytopenia, microangiopathic hemolytic anemia, increased LDH levels, fever, transient neurologic deficits and renal failure.*
- *This is due to widespread hyaline microthrombi found in arterioles and capillaries.*
- *Peak incidence is in third decade of life and female are more affected.*
- *Pathogenesis: Deficiency of VWF or antibodies to metalloprotease ADAMTS 13 that cleaves VWF.*
- *The presence of severe Coomb's negative hemolytic anemia with fragmented RBC in peripheral smear, thrombocytopenia and minimal activation of coagulation **confirms** the diagnosis.*
- *TTP is treated with corticosteroids, platelet aggregation inhibitors and exchange transfusion.*
- *Plasma exchange (also called plasmapheresis) is used to treat acquired TTP.*
  - o *This is a lifesaving procedure.*
  - o *It **removes** antibodies (proteins) from the blood that damage ADAMTS 13 enzyme.*
  - o *Plasma exchange also replaces the ADAMTS 13 enzyme.*

- *Platelet infusion is contraindicated because it promotes micro-thrombi formation.*

Coming back to the question:

- *Plasmapheresis in thrombotic thrombocytopenic purpura acts by removing anti-ADAMTS13 antibodies.*

12. An old male was brought to the Medicine OPD by his son. His son says that his father do not use his left side arm and leg. He also do not clean the left side of his body. A diagram was given to the patient (left side images) to copy and his drawing is also shown (right side of images). Such a manifestation could be because of lesion in:

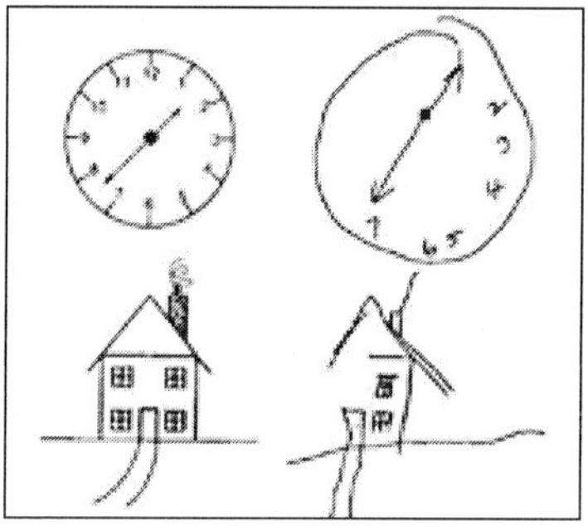

A. Right motor cortex
B. Left motor cortex
C. Right posterior parietal cortex
D. Left posterior parietal cortex

Clinical presentation is indicative of left hemispatial neglect.

Key points about Hemispatial neglect:

- *It results **most** commonly from strokes and brain unilateral injury to the **right** cerebral hemisphere, with rates in the critical stage of up to 80% causing visual neglect of the left-hand side of space.*
- *Neglect is often produced by massive strokes in the middle cerebral artery region and is variegated, so that **most** sufferers do **not** exhibit all of the syndrome traits.*
- *Although it **most** strikingly affects visual perception ('visual neglect'), neglect in other forms of perception can also be found, either alone or in combination with visual neglect.*

- *For example, a stroke affecting the right parietal lobe of the brain can lead to neglect for the left side of the visual field, causing a patient with neglect to behave as if the left side of sensory space is non-existent (although they can still turn left).*
- *In an extreme case, a patient with neglect might fail to eat the food on the left half of their plate, even though they complain of being hungry.*
- *If someone with neglect is asked to draw a* **clock**, *their drawing might show only the numbers 12 to 6, or all 12 numbers might be on one half of the clock face with the other half distorted or blank.*
- *Neglect patients may also ignore the contralesional side of their body; for instance, they might only shave, or apply make-up to, the non-neglected side.*
- *These patients may frequently collide with objects or structures such as door frames on the side being neglected.*
- *Brain areas in the parietal and frontal lobes are associated with the deployment of attention (internally, or through eye movements, head turns or limb reaches) into contralateral space.*
- *Neglect is* **most** *closely related to damage to the temporoparietal junction and* **posterior parietal** *cortex.*

Let's discuss the options:

Option	*Statement*	*Remarks*
a	Right motor cortex	• Lesions of the right sided pre-central gyrus result in paralysis of the left side of the body (facial palsy, arm/leg monoparesis, hemiparesis); UMN lesion.
b	Left motor cortex	• Lesions of the left sided pre-central gyrus result in paralysis of the right side of the body (facial palsy, arm/leg monoparesis, hemiparesis); UMN lesion.
c	Right posterior parietal cortex	• Lesions of right posterior parietal cortex results in left-sided spatial neglect.

Contd.

d	Left posterior parietal cortex	• Lesions of left posterior parietal cortex does **not** cause right-sided spatial neglect because there is redundant processing of the right space by both the left and right cerebral hemispheres.

Coming back to the question:

- *A person with left hemi neglect will not use his left side arm and leg. He will not clean left side of his body. When he is asked to copy an image, he will draw only the right part of the image and will not draw the left half of the given image. Left hemi neglect is seen with involvement of right posterior parietal cortex.*

13. Calculate the anion gap from the given set of values:

Na^+: 145 mEq/L, K^+: 4 mEq/L, Cl^-: 90 mEq/L and HCO_3: 20 mmol/L

A. 12 mmol/L
B. 28 mmol/L
C. 35 mmol/L
D. 44 mmol/L

Key points about Anion gap:

- *The number of cations and anions in the body fluids are equal and neutralize each other.*
- *Sodium, potassium, calcium and magnesium are the cations.*
- *Bicarbonate, chloride, sulphate, phosphate, organic acid and albumin are the anions.*
- *Only sodium, bicarbonate and chloride are taken into consideration for the calculation of anion gap.*
- *Anion gap = $Na^+ - (HCO_3^- + Cl^-)$.*
- *The gap consists of the anions that are usually not measured or included in the calculation.*
- *The normal value of anion gap is approximately 12 ± 2 mmol/L.*
- *For the purpose of calculation of anion gap, unmeasured anions (UA) and unmeasured cations (UC) and potassium are discarded.*

Coming back to the question:

- *Anion gap = $Na^+ - (HCO_3^- + Cl^-) = 145 - (90 + 20) = 35$ mmol/L.*

14. A young female presented to the Emergency room with the complaints of palpitation. She develops syncope and becomes hypotensive. ECG was done as shown below. Most likely diagnosis:

A. Monomorphic ventricular tachycardia
B. Ventricular fibrillation
C. Atrial fibrillation
D. Torsade de pointes

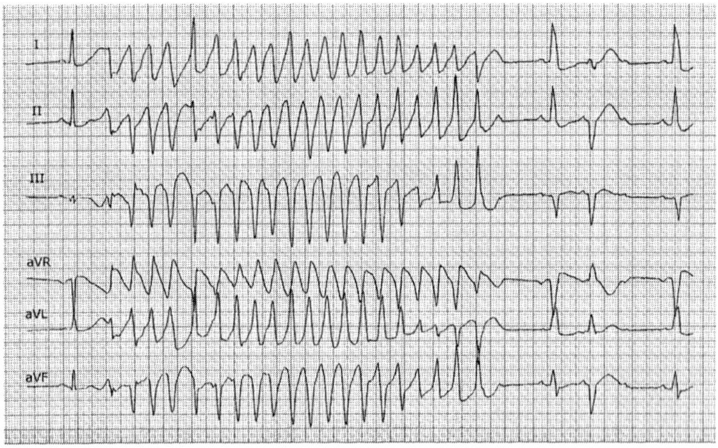

Let's discuss the options:

Option	*Statement*	*Remarks*
a	Monomorphic Ventricular tachycardia	• Three or more successive ventricular premature complexes are termed ventricular tachycardia/VT. • Classic monomorphic VT means VT with **uniform** QRS complexes morphology throughout the arrhythmia. • Indeterminate axis. • Very broad QRS (nearly 200 ms).

Contd.

b	Ventricular fibrillation	• VF occurs in various clinical situations but is **most** commonly associated with coronary artery disease and as a terminal event. • It is **most** commonly identified arrhythmia in cardiac arrest patients. • On ECG, VF is recognized by the presence of irregular undulations of varying contour and amplitude.
c	Atrial fibrillation	• Ventricular rate may be slow, normal or fast; atrial rate is greater than 350 beats per minute. • Totally irregular (chaotic). • P waves are **absent**; instead there is a chaotic-looking baseline. • QRS complexes are normal. • PR interval is absent.
d	Torsade de pointes	• Ventricular flutter may present with multiform QRS complexes, a manifestation which has been termed 'TdP'. • In this presentation, the QRS complexes tend to be bizarre and multiform, and have sharply **pointed** apices or nadirs. • This form of ventricular flutter is likely to complicate advanced and third stage AV block, and is frequently associated with **syncopal** attacks. • The syncopal attacks may result in marked prolongation of the QT_c interval and there may be 'giant T-wave inversion'.

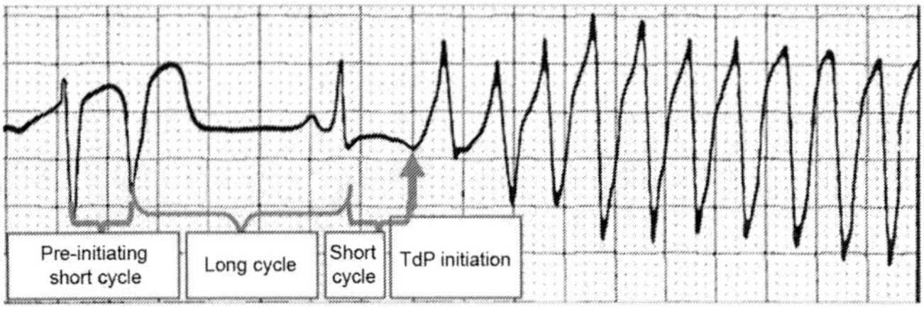

Coming back to the question:

- *Torsade de pointes is a polymorphic ventricular tachycardia in the range of 180-250 beats/min characterized by QRS complexes of progressively changing amplitude and contour, that seem to revolve around the isoelectric line.*

15. Identify the clinical sign elicited in the given image:

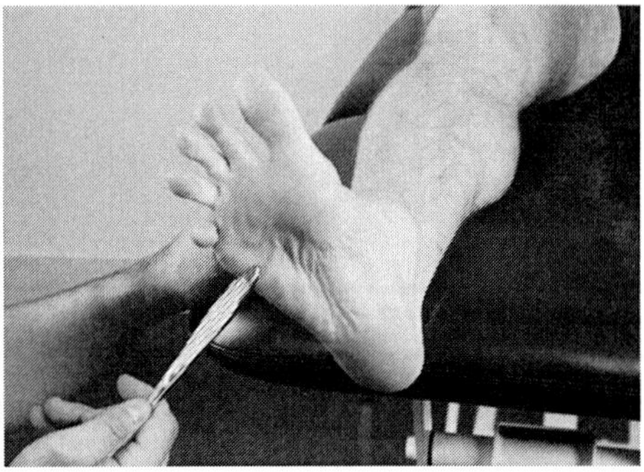

A. Ankle clonus
B. Hoffman reflex
C. Babinski's sign
D. Oppenheim reflex

Let's discuss the options:

Option	*Statement*	*Remarks*
a	Ankle clonus	• Sudden stretching of hypertonic muscles produces reflex contraction. • If stretched is maintained during the subsequent relaxation, further reflex contraction occurs and this may continue almost indefinitely, unless the stretch stimulus is released.

Contd.

		• It is most easily demonstrated by dorsiflexing the foot, after flexing the hip and knee (ankle clonus) or by sharply moving the patella downwards (patellar clonus).
b	Hoffman reflex	• The terminal phalanx of the patient's middle finger is flicked downwards between the examiner's finger and thumb. • In states of hypertonia, the tips of the other fingers flex and thumb flexes and adducts.
c	Babinski sign	• It is also known as extensor plantar response. • This response is seen with lesions of the corticospinal tract (pyramidal tract). • On eliciting the plantar response, there is dorsiflexion of the great toe, along with extension and fanning out of the other toes. • In addition, especially if the response is marked, there is dorsiflexion at the ankle, with flexion at the knee and hip, these associated movements being bought about by the contraction of the anterior tibial, hamstrings, and tensor fascia lata.
d	Oppenheim reflex	• It is another method of obtaining plantar reflex. • A form stroke with the finger and thumb is applied down either side of the anterior border of the tibia, greater pressure being applied to the medial side.

Coming back to the question:

- *The clinical sign elicited in the given image is Babinski's sign.*

16. A 55 years old woman presented with daytime sleepiness and memory loss for the last 1 year. Her blood pressure is 170/98 mm of Hg and BMI is 43. Awake arterial blood gas analysis showed pO_2 of 70 mm Hg, $paCO_2$ of 53 mm Hg and HCO_3^- of 33 mmol/L. Most likely diagnosis:

A. Obstructive sleep apnea
B. Central sleep apnea
C. Obesity hypoventilation syndrome
D. Narcolepsy

Let's discuss the options:

Option	*Statement*	*Remarks*
a	Obstructive sleep apnea/OSA	• The cessation of breathing may be due to occlusion of the airway.
b	Central sleep apnea/CSA	• CSA is characterized by a **lack** of drive to breather during sleep, resulting in insufficient or absent ventilation and compromised gas exchange. • In contrast to OSA, in which ongoing respiratory efforts are observed, CSA is defined by lack of respiratory efforts during cessation of airflow. • Considerable overlap exists in the pathogenesis and pathophysiology of OSA and CSA, making this distinction somewhat difficult at times. • CSA, like OSA, is associated with important complications, including frequent night time awakenings, excessive day time sleepiness, and increased risk of adverse cardiovascular outcomes. • Typically, CSA is considered to the primary diagnosis when ≥50% of the apneas are scored as central in origin (i.e., >10 seconds cessation

Contd.

		of breathing in the absence of respiratory effort). • CSA syndromes can be broadly classified into two groups according to the wakefulness CO_2 levels (hypercapnic and non-hypercapnic).
c	Obesity hypoventilation syndrome/OHS	• One of the form of hypercapnic CSA is OHS. • The disorder is typically defined as a combination of **obesity** (body mass index >30 kg/m^2) and arterial **hyper-capnia** ($paCO_2$ >45 mm Hg) during wakefulness not explained by other known causes of hypoventilation. • Hypoventilation worsens during non-REM sleep and further during REM sleep, resulting in marked hypercapnia with accompanying **hypoxemia**. • Typical symptoms may be similar to patients with OSA, including morning headaches and daytime hypersomnolence.
d	Narcolepsy	• There is excessive daytime sleepiness with involuntary daytime sleep episodes, disturbed nocturnal sleep and cataplexy (sudden weakness or loss of muscle tone often elicited by emotion). • It consists of clinical tetrad of: o Excessive daytime somnolence. o Cataplexy. o Hypnogogic hallucinations. o Sleep paralysis.

Coming back to the question:

- *Daytime sleepiness, BMI of 43, ABG showing pO_2 of 70 mm Hg and $PaCO_2$ of 53 mm Hg, suggest the diagnosis of obesity hypoventilation syndrome.*

17. In a case of aortic insufficiency, the murmur is likely to be heard:

A. During rapid filling phase
B. During isovolumetric relaxation phase
C. During isovolumetric contraction phase
D. Throughout the cardiac cycle

Key points about murmur in AR:

- *A high frequency decrescendo* ***early diastolic*** *murmur/EDM is heard immediately after A2.*
- *It is best heard in left 3rd and 4th spaces with the diaphragm of the stethoscope with the patient leaning forwards, in expiration.*

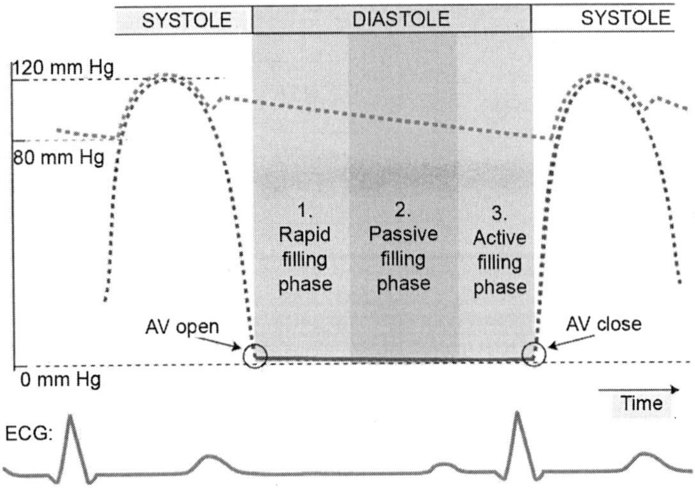

Coming back to the question:

- *In aortic regurgitation, a murmur is heard in early diastole, which corresponds to rapid filling phase of the ventricular diastole.*

SURGERY

1. A patient has been vomiting severely since last 2 days. He developed orthostatic hypotension too. Which of the following will be seen in such a patient?

I. Hypokalemia
II. Hyponatremia
III. Hypochloremia
IV. Respiratory alkalosis

Lead – Choose the best answer from the codes given below:

A. I and II
B. II and III
C. I, II and III
D. I, II, III and IV

Key points about Electrolyte changes in severe vomiting:

- *The vomiting of gastric or intestinal contents most commonly involves the loss of fluid that contains chloride, potassium and sodium.*
- *The sequelae of these loses include dehydration along with hyponatremia, hypochloremia, hypocalcemia, hypomagnesemia and hypokalemia.*
- *The removal of gastric HCl due to vomiting results in* ***metabolic*** *alkalosis because bicarbonate is added to the ECF (rather than secreted into the small bowel lumen).*

Coming back to the question:

- *Severe vomiting causes hypochloremic, hyponatremic, hypokalemic, hypocalcemic, hypomagnesemic, metabolic alkalosis.*

2. Match the following:

Structure involved in thyroid swelling	***Symptoms***
1. Trachea	**A. Dysphagia**
2. Esophagus	**B. Hoarseness of voice**
3. Recurrent laryngeal nerve	**C. Dyspnea**
4. Sympathetic chain	**D. Horner's syndrome**

Lead – Choose the best answer from the codes given below:

A. 1-B, 2-A, 3-D, 4-C
B. 1-C, 2-B, 3-A, 4-D
C. 1-A, 2-B, 3-C, 4-D
D. 1-C, 2-A, 3-B, 4-D

Let's discuss the options:

Option	*Statement*	*Remarks*
1	Trachea	• Tracheal compression may cause cough, stridor, **dyspnea** or orthopnea.
2	Esophagus	• The most frequent symptoms related to extrinsic esophageal compression is mechanical **dysphagia**, first for solids and in cases of advanced obstruction, for liquids as well.
3	Recurrent laryngeal nerve	• Injury to the recurrent laryngeal nerve has the potential to cause unilateral vocal cord paralysis. • Patients with this typically complain of new-onset **hoarseness**, changes in vocal pitch, or noisy breathing.
4	Sympathetic chain	• **Horner's** syndrome/Oculosympathetic paresis results from an interruption of the sympathetic nerve supply to the eye and is characterized by the classic triad of miosis, partial ptosis and loss of hemifacial sweating, as well as enophthalmos.

Coming back to the question:

Condition	*Feature*
1. Trachea	*C. Dyspnea*
2. Esophagus	*A. Dysphagia*
3. Recurrent laryngeal nerve	*B. Hoarseness of voice*
4. Sympathetic chain	*D. Horner's syndrome*

3. Identify the condition shown below:

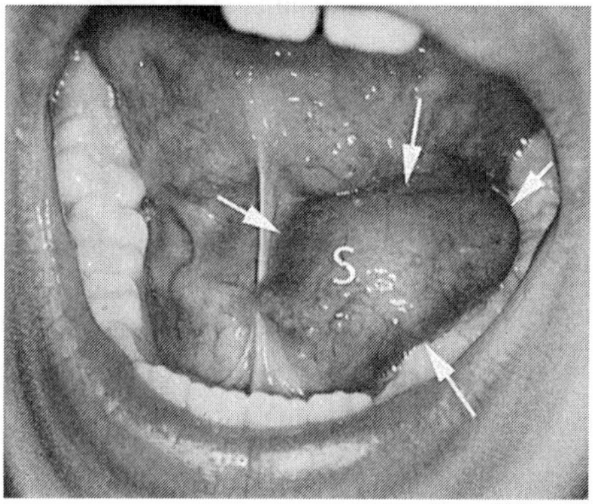

A. Epidermoid cyst
B. Ranula
C. Cystic hygroma
D. Branchial cyst

Let's discuss the options:

Option	*Statement*	*Remarks*
a	Epidermoid cyst	• Epidermoid cyst/Sebaceous cyst is a retention cyst. • It is due to the blockage of the duct of sebaceous gland, causing a cystic swelling. • Sebaceous glands are situated in dermic which secretes sebum through sebaceous ducts which open either directly to skin surface or into a hair follicle. • It is **common** in face, scalp, scrotum. • It is **not** seen in palms and soles as there are no sebaceous glands. • It presents as a painless swelling which is smooth, soft, non-tender, freely mobile, adherent to skin especially over the summit, fluctuant (positive Paget's test), **non**-transilluminating with punctum over the summit.

Contd.

b	Ranula	• Ranula looks like belly of frog, hence the name (Rana = Frog). • Ranula is an extravasation cyst arising from sublingual gland or mucous glands of Nuhn or glands of Blandin in the floor of the mouth. • Initially there is blockage of the duct (of sublingual gland) causing retention cyst, which causes rupture of the acini due to increased pressure leading into extravasation cyst. • It presents as a bluish smooth, soft, fluctuant, brilliantly transilluminant swelling in the lateral aspect of the floor of the mouth.
c	Cystic hygroma	• Also known as cavernous hemangioma/ hydrocele of the neck. • It is a cystic swelling due to sequestration of a portion of jugular lymph sac from the lymphatic system, during the development period in utero. • Present at birth (in the posterior triangle of the neck) and so may cause obstructed labour. • Swelling is smooth, non-tender, soft, fluctuant (cystic), partially compressible, brilliantly transilluminant. • It is **not** reducible completely. • During crying swelling often increases in size. • Swelling may rapidly increase in size causing respiratory obstruction – **dangerous** sign.
d	Branchial cyst	• It arises from the remnants of second branchial cleft. • Normally 2nd, 3rd, 4th clefts disappear to form a smooth neck.

Contd.

		• Persistent 2nd cleft is called as cervical sinus (of His) which eventually gets sequestrated to form branchial cyst. • Swelling in the neck beneath the anterior border of upper third of sternomastoid muscle. • It is smooth, soft, fluctuant, often transilluminant with a sensation of 'Half-filled double hot water bottle'. • Usually painless unless it is infected. • It contains cholesterol crystals which is from the lining of mucous membrane which contains sebaceous gland. • Cheesy toothpaste like material is **typical**.

Coming back to the question:

- *Ranula presents as a laterally placed, bluish swelling in the floor of the mouth.*

4. All of the following are perineal procedures for rectal prolapse EXCEPT:

A. Delorme operation B. Thiersch wiring
C. Ripstein operation D. Altemeier rectosigmoidectomy

Let's discuss the options:

Option	***Statement***	***Remarks***
a	Delorme operation	• Perineal procedure (Mucosal sleeve resection and plication). • After bowel preparation, under spinal anesthesia, in lithotomy position, completely prolapsed rectum is held with Babcock's forceps. • 1 in 2,00,000 adrenaline solution is injected into the submucosal plane of the rectum to cause hemostasis.

Contd.

		• By making longitudinal incision, with sharp scissor and cautery dissection, mucosa is stripped off from the deeper muscular layer from 1 cm below the anal margin to the apex of the prolapse rectum. • Muscular layer of rectum is plicated using absorbable vicryl 2 zero interrupted sutures all around; approximately 12-15 plication stitches are needed. • These sutures are tied after finishing the passage of all sutures. • Cut end of the mucosa of the apex is sutured to anal margin using interrupted vicryl sutures.
b	Thiersch wiring	• Perineal procedure. • In 1891, Thiersch did anal encircling using silver wire to provoke inflammatory fibrosis as well as to give mechanical support to the anal orifice – Thiersch wiring. • It is done under local anesthesia. • Two small incisions are made at lateral parts of the anal canal. • Silver wire is passed around deeper to these incisions and tied after placing the index finger into the anal canal. • Wire can be removed after 12 months.
c	Ripstein operation	• **Abdominal** procedure. • After mobilization of the rectum, 5 cm width Teflon mesh sling is passed around the rectum to fix it behind to fascia 5 cm below and in front of the sacral promontory. • Sling is also fixed in front and laterally to rectum.

Contd.

d	Altemeier recto-sigmoidectomy	• Perineal procedure. • After rectosigmoidectomy, colonic anastomosis and pelvic floor is supported by suturing in front of the rectum using non-absorbable sutures.

Coming back to the question:

- *Ripstein operation for rectal prolapse is an abdominal procedure.*

5. Identify the type of hernia shown in the image:

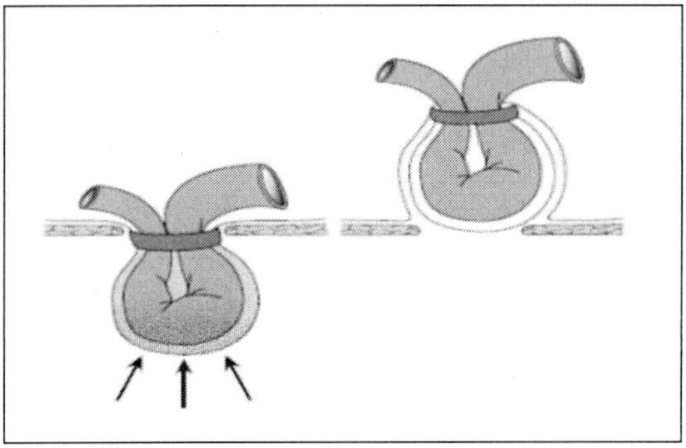

A. Incarcerated hernia
B. Reduction en masse
C. Sliding hernia
D. Maydl's hernia

Let's discuss the options:

Option	*Statement*	*Remarks*
a	Incarcerated hernia	• Here the lumen of the portion of colon occupying a hernia sac is blocked with feces. • Here scybalous content of the bowel should be capable of being indented with the finger, like putty. • In incarcerated hernia, sac and contents are densely adherent to each other (contents are fixed to sac). • It is **always** irreducible; often obstructed but may not be strangulated.

Contd.

b	Reduction en masse	• In an obstructed hernia, if reduction is forced, it may get reduced with the sac and ring with the obstructed/ strangulated bowel. • Reduction en masse may **mask** the gangrenous bowel existing in the sac.
c	Sliding hernia	• Hernia-en-glissade. • Here part of the posterior wall formed is **not** only by the parietal peritoneum but also by part of retroperitoneal structures. • **Most** common on left side (85%). • **Most** common content overall (and on left side): Sigmoid colon with its mesentery. • **Most** common content on right side: Cecum. • Presents as large globular swelling in the inguinal region descending into the scrotum, often irreducible. • During surgery, do **not** dissect the sac from the retroperitoneal structures, just push part of the sac along with them. • If tried, injury may result to these organs leading to fecal or urinary fistulas.
d	Maydl's hernia	• Hernia-in-W. • Here a loop of bowel in the form of 'W' lies in the hernia sac and the centre portion of the 'W' loop is strangulated and lies within the abdominal cavity. • Thus local tenderness over the hernia is not marked and hernia gets reduced with the strangulated loop in the centre of the 'W'. • Strangulation in this case is often missed during surgery and may lead to peritonitis due to retained gangrenous loops.

Coming back to the question:

- *In Reduction en masse, if reduction is forced in an obstructed hernia, it may get reduced with the sac and ring with the obstructed/ strangulated bowel.*

6. Identify the instrument shown below:

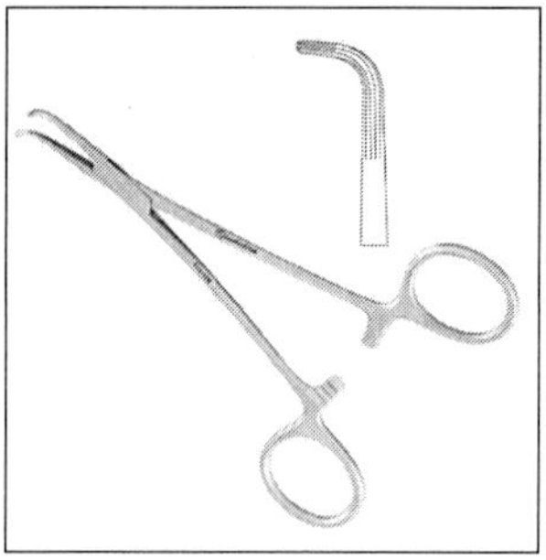

A. Morrant-Baker's forceps
B. Allis' forceps
C. Mixter forceps
D. Babcock's forceps

Let's discuss the options:

Option	*Statement*	*Remarks*
a	Morrant-Baker's forceps	• It is also known as appendix holding forceps. • It has apposing serration proximal to the tooth. • These serrations give a good grip in mesoappendix while holding the appendix in appendicectomy. • Its use is replaced by Babcock's forceps.
b	Allis' forceps	• It is also known as tissue holding forceps. • Here distal blades are not apposing each other. • Tip has got teeth in each blade which are apposing. • It has got a lock on the proximal part. • It is used to hold skin flaps, fasciae, aponeurosis, bladder wall.

Contd.

c	Mixter forceps	• Mixter hemostatic forceps are versatile surgery instruments used to clamp the blood vessels and prevent blood loss. • They are used to control bleeding from the blood vessels. • Overall instrument length is $5^{1/4}$ inch and features a delicate pattern along with half serrated jaws that are slightly curved.
d	Babcock's forceps	• Its distal part of the distal blades is curved with a triangular fenestra in it which allow soft tissues to bulge out. • Tip is non-traumatic with transverse serrations on it. • It has got a lock in the proximal part. • It is used to hold any part of the bowel, fallopian tubes, appendix, ureter, cord, etc.

Coming back to the question:

- *Mixter forceps are used to control bleeding from the vessels.*

7. Which of the following tests are done to check saphenofemoral junction incompetence?

I. Trendelenburg test I

II. Morrissey cough impulse test

III. Fegan's test

IV. Perthes test

Lead – Choose the best answer from the codes given below:

A. I and II
B. II and III
C. I, II and III
D. I, II, III and IV

Let's discuss the options:

Option	*Statement*	*Remarks*
I	Trendelenburg test I	• Vein is emptied by elevating the limb and a tourniquet is tied just below the saphenofemoral junction/SFJ (or using thumb, SFJ is occluded).

Contd.

		• Patient is asked to stand quickly. • When tourniquet or thumb is released, rapid filling from above signifies saphenofemoral **incompetence**.
II	Morrissey cough impulse test	• The varicose veins are emptied. • The leg is elevated and the patient is asked to cough. • If there is saphenofemoral **incompetence**, expansile impulse is felt at saphenous opening. • It is a venous thrill due to vibration caused by turbulent backflow.
III	Fegan's test	• On standing, the site where the perforators enter the deep fascia bulges and this is marked. • Then on lying down, button like depression (crescent like) in the deep fascia is felt at the marked out points which confirms the **perforator** site.
IV	Perthes test	• The affected lower limb is wrapped with elastic bandage and the patient is asked to walk around and exercise. • Development of severe cramp like pain in the calf signifies deep venous thrombosis/**DVT**.

Coming back to the question:

- *Trendelenburg test I and Morrissey's cough impulse test checks saphenofemoral incompetence.*

8. Smoking is a risk factor for the development of:

I. Duct ectasia | **II. Mondor's disease**

III. Carcinoma breast | **IV. Fibroadenoma**

Lead – Choose the best answer from the codes given below:

A. I and II | B. II and III

C. I, II and III | D. I, II, III and IV

Let's discuss the options:

Option	*Statement*	*Remarks*
I	Duct ectasia	• Duct ectasia is dilatation of lactiferous ducts due to muscular relaxation (myoepithelial relaxation) of duct wall with periductal mastitis. • Cigarette **smoking** may be associated with widening of milk ducts, which can lead to inflammation and, possibly, mammary duct ectasia.
II	Mondor's disease	• Mondor's disease is spontaneous thrombophlebitis of the superficial veins of the breast and anterior chest wall. • As **smoking** is one of the factors that induce coagulatory processes and Mondor's disease is characterized by thrombophlebitis of veins, this may be a reasonable hypothesis.
III	Carcinoma breast	• Women who are current smokers and have been **smoking** for more than 10 years appear to have about a 10% higher risk of breast cancer than women who have never smoked.
IV	Fibroadenoma	• It is a benign encapsulated tumour occurring commonly in young females of 15-25 years' age group. • Presently it is considered as hyperplasia of a single lobule of the breast (classified under ANDI). • It is **A**berration in **N**ormal **D**evelopment (**AND**) of a lobule. • It is the **most** common benign tumour of the breast below 30 years of age in females. • It does **not** turn into malignancy.

Coming back to the question:

- *Smoking is a risk factor for development of duct ectasia, Mondor's disease and carcinoma breast.*

9. All of the following are true for breast conservation surgery EXCEPT:

A. Sentinel lymph node biopsy/SLNB is done
B. Frozen section is needed
C. Radiotherapy is not needed post-operatively
D. Wide local excision and axillary dissection is done

Key points about Wide local excision:

- *It is a type of conservative breast surgery.*
- *It is removal of unicentric tumour with 1 cm clearance margin.*
- *Incision is made directly over the tumour.*
- *Skin flaps should **not** be raised.*
- *Normal breast tissue of 1 cm clearance with excision of tumour is done.*
- *Pectoral fascia is usually **not** opened in wide local excision unlike in total mastectomy.*
- *The specimen is marked after placing in orientation grid and mammography of the specimen is done followed by **frozen** section biopsy to look for clearance.*
- *At least 1 mm clearance is needed for adequacy.*
- *Margins where clearance is less 1 mm need re-excision at that particular margin.*
- *If margins show **no** clearance, then patient requires probably total mastectomy.*
- *So prior consent for mastectomy should be taken.*
- *Drain is **not** placed; deeper cavity is usually **not** closed/obliterated as small seroma gets absorbed without any problem.*
- *Skin is closed cosmetically.*
- *It is often called as lumpectomy or partial mastectomy; but the term is **wide** local excision.*
- *It is ideal breast conservative surgery.*
- *Along with this, **axillary** dissection through separate incision and **radiotherapy** to breast and chest wall is given.*
- *Wide local excision of the primary tumour is done after **SLNB** in the same sitting.*

Coming back to the question:

- *Radiotherapy to the breast tissue and chest wall is given after wide local excision.*

10. An elderly male presented with bleeding per rectum. All of the following investigations are done in such a case EXCEPT:

I. CT scan
II. CA 19-9
III. Colonoscopy
IV. Carcinoembryonic antigen

Lead – Choose the best answer from the codes given below:

A. I and II
B. II and III
C. I, II and III
D. I, III and IV

Clinical presentation is indicative of colorectal carcinoma.

Let's discuss the options:

Option	*Statement*	*Remarks*
I	CT scan	• CT scan abdomen and pelvis is done in colorectal carcinoma to see local spread, invasion, size and extent, stage, nodal status and liver secondaries.
II	CA 19-9	• Carbohydrate antigen 19-9, first described in 1979, is a cell surface glycoprotein complex produced by ductal cells in the pancreas, biliary system, and epithelial cells in some parts of GIT. • CA 19-9 is overexpressed in many benign and malignant, gastrointestinal and extra-gastrointestinal diseases. • Its main implications are in **pancreatic** ductal adenocarcinoma and intraductal papillary mucinous neoplasm (IPMN).
III	Colonoscopy	• Colonoscopy is the **most** accurate and **most** complete method for evaluating the entire colon in colorectal carcinoma.

Contd.

		• It allows identification of small polyps (<1 cm), allows biopsy, polypectomy, control of bleeding, stricture dilatation if needed. • Problem as a screening method is – prior need for mechanical bowel preparation.
IV	Carcino-embryonic antigen	• Pre-operative levels of CEA >7.5 ng/ml signify **poor** prognosis in colorectal carcinoma. • If postoperative level does **not** fall, it indicates either incomplete resection, or occult metastasis elsewhere. • Increase CEA during follow-up indicates recurrence or secondaries. • A slow rise indicates loco regional disease. • A rapid rise signifies metastasis. • It is **not** useful in assessing follow-up in poorly differentiated adenocarcinoma as such tumour will not produce CEA.

Coming back to the question:

- *CA 19-9 is not included in the diagnostic workup of colorectal carcinoma.*

11. All of the following are complications of Total Parenteral Nutrition/TPN EXCEPT:

A. Osteoporosis   B. Refeeding syndrome
C. Pneumothorax   D. Aspiration

Key points about TPN:

- *All nutritional requirements are given only through intravenous route, not through gastrointestinal tract.*
- *It can be through a central catheter through the Subclavian/Internal jugular vein where the tip of venous catheter is at distal part of superior vena cava.*

- *Technical complications:*
  - *Air embolism.*
  - ***Pneumothorax**.*
  - *Bleeding.*
  - *Catheter displacement, sepsis, blockage.*
- *Biochemical complications:*
  - *Electrolyte imbalance: Hyponatremia, hypokalemia, hypophosphatemia.*
  - *Hyperosmolarity.*
  - *Hyperglycemia – **common**.*
  - *Dehydration.*
  - *Azotemia.*
- ***Refeeding** syndrome:*
  - *It is occurrence of severe fluid and electrolyte imbalance in severely malnourished individual while starting the proper feeding enteral or parenteral nutrition.*
  - *It is **more** common in TPN.*
  - *It causes hypomagnesemia, **hypocalcemia** and hypophosphatemia.*
- *Other complications:*
  - *Dermatitis.*
  - *Cholestatic jaundice – It is **common**.*
  - *Severe hepatic steatosis.*
  - *Metabolic acidosis.*
  - *Candidiasis.*

Coming back to the question:

- *Aspiration is not a complication of TPN as nothing is given by mouth.*

12. A young male patient presented with mild fever and pain in right upper abdominal quadrant for last 7 days. There is past history of dysentery 6 weeks back. CT scan showed a hypoechoic lesion with irregular border as shown below. Most likely diagnosis:

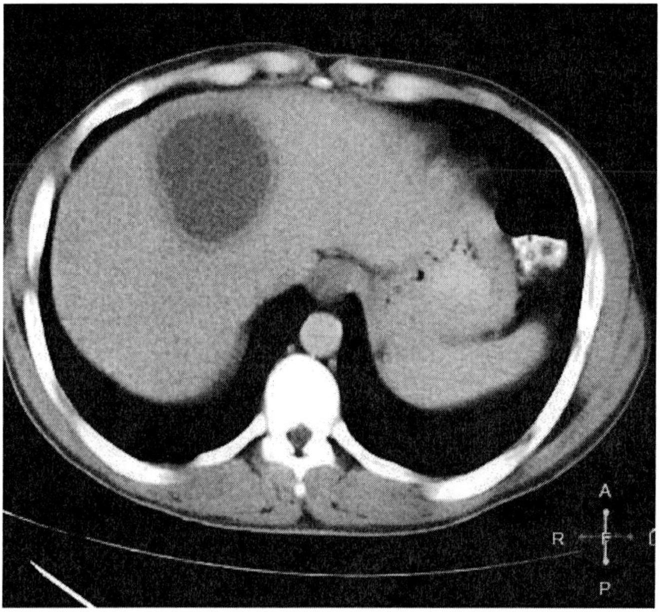

A. Hydatid disease of liver
B. Amoebic liver abscess
C. Pyogenic liver abscess
D. Hemangioma of liver

Let's discuss the options:

Option	*Statement*	*Remarks*
a	Hydatid disease of liver	• Patient may present with jaundice and pain. • Asymptomatic palpable liver with **classical** thrill (hydatid thrill) elicited by three-finger test. • Feature of anaphylaxis. • Discomfort in the right upper quadrant area; dyspepsia; hydatid cachexia in children; weight loss; fatigue. • CT scan abdomen is **more** accurate in identifying cyst characteristics – cart wheel like – multivesicular rosette like.

Contd.

b	Amoebic liver abscess	• It is **more** common in **males** (10:1), may be after an attack of amoebic **dysentery** or many months after the attack or history of dysentery may **not** be there at all. • They present with **fever**, loss of weight, chills and rigors, non-productive cough, shoulder pain. • **Pain** in the right hypochondrium – 90%. • Soft, tender, smooth, liver with increased liver span – 70%. • Intercostal tenderness is elicited which is a **useful** clinical sign. • CT scan-contrast study shows raised diaphragm; abscess cavity (**low** density area) – its size, location, number, presence of effusion; changes in the lung – 95% sensitivity.
c	Pyogenic liver abscess	• Biliary sepsis 35%; **most common** route. • Usually solitary – 60%. • Pain in the right hypochondrium – 60% cases. • **High** fever, with rigors – 90%. • Weight loss. • Jaundice – occasionally – 20%. • Tender, soft liver – 60%. • Sensitivity is 97% for contrast CT scan.
d	Hemangioma of liver	• Hemangiomas are the most common benign tumour of the liver. • It is usually solitary but can be multi-centric. • Compressibility of the tumour is **diagnostic**. • It is **common** in females (3:1) in 5th decade. • Commonly they are asymptomatic. • They can occur in right and left lobes. • CT scan is confirmative.

Coming back to the question:

- *In a young male patient, mild fever and pain in right upper abdominal quadrant with a past history of dysentery suggest the diagnosis of amoebic liver abscess.*

13. Identify the condition shown in the image:

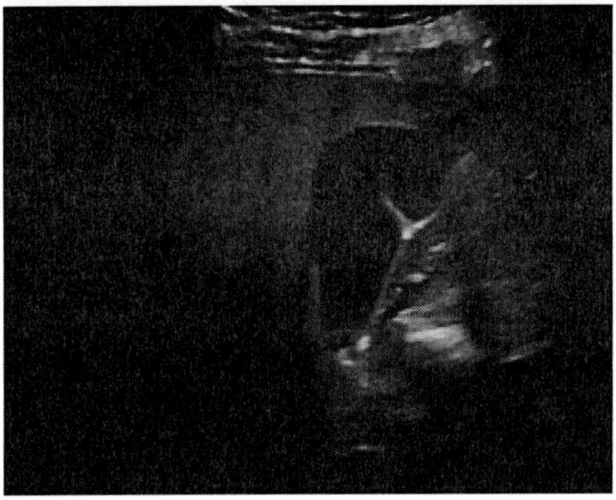

A. Gallbladder polyp
B. Gallbladder carcinoma
C. Phrygian cap
D. Floating gallbladder

Let's discuss the options:

Option	*Statement*	*Remarks*
a	Gallbladder polyp	• Its incidence is 5% in routine USG abdomen; 10% in cholecystectomy tissue specimen. • It is usually less than 10 mm in size, pedunculated appearance. • **USG** features: A non-shadowing polypoid ingrowth into the gallbladder lumen, which is usually immobile unless there is a relatively long pedunculated component. • Gallbladder polyp more than 10 mm in size, associated with gallstones, age above 60 years, symptomatic, sessile polyp and multiple polyps – are indications for surgical intervention.

Contd.

b	Gallbladder carcinoma	• In carcinoma gallbladder, USG can depict a focal intraluminal, wall involvement, or large mass-like lesion replacing the gallbladder. • The tumour usually has irregular and sometimes ill-defined margins, with heterogeneous echotexture and predominantly low echogenicity. • Hyperechoic foci with posterior acoustic shadowing may be seen within the mass, possibly reflecting gallstones or gallbladder wall calcifications (porcelain gallbladder).
c	Phrygian cap	• Cap like projection and bend over the fundus of the gallbladder (Phrygia is an ancient Asian country - Mongolia) (Liberty cap of French revolution). • It is identified in cholecystogram. • It is 6% common. • May be **wrongly** interpreted as a septum in an otherwise normal gallbladder.
d	Floating gallbladder	• Mobile/floating/mesenteric gallbladder has a long mesentery attached. • It may cause torsion. • It can cause recurrent abdominal pain. • Its removal is easier through laparoscopic or open method.

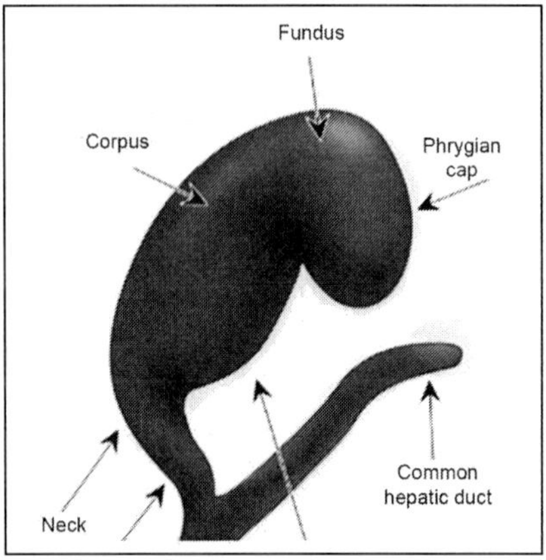

Coming back to the question:

- *Phrygian cap denotes folding of the fundus back upon the gallbladder body (corpus).*

14. All of the following are advantages of USG over mammography EXCEPT:

A. USG can be used for palpable breast mass which are mammographically undetectable
B. USG is helpful in young females
C. USG guided FNAC can be performed
D. USG can differentiate between solid and cystic breast lesions

Key points about USG of breast:

- *To look for whether the lesion is solid or **cystic**, margin of the lesion, internal echoes, retro tumour acoustic, shadowing, compressibility, dimensions.*
- *Irregular margin, irregular internal echoes, irregular posterior shadowing, noncompressibility, ratio between anteroposterior to width (lateral/horizontal) dimensions more than 1 are the **features** of carcinoma. Doppler will show high frequency signals with continuous flow. It is hypoechoic with more vertical taller growth.*
- *Benign lesions are smooth, rounded with well-defined margins with weak internal echoes and compressibility. It can be elliptical, hyperechoic/hypoechoic smooth lesion.*
- *Cyst is anechoic, oval/round, well circumscribed lesion.*
- *Disadvantage is lesions less than 1 cm may **not** be identified.*
- ***FNAC** can be done under USG guidance.*
- *It is cheaper, easily available and there is **no** risk of radiation.*
- *It is **preferred** method of screening in **young** females where mammography is **not** done and in pregnancy and early lactation.*
- *USG of axilla also can be done to assess axilla and to do guided FNAC of the lymph node.*

Coming back to the question:

- *Lesions indeterminate by mammography are best assessed by MRI, so USG cannot be used for palpable breast mass which are mammographically undetectable.*

15. A 30 years old male presented with abdominal pain, fatigue and dysuria. X-ray abdomen was done as shown below. Most likely diagnosis:

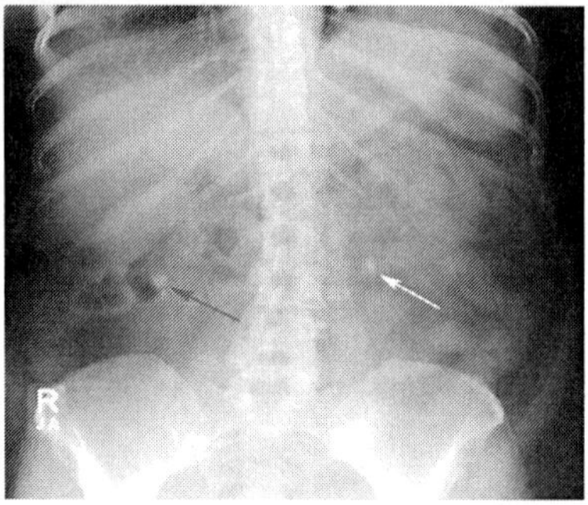

A. Ankylosing spondylitis
B. Perforated peptic ulcer
C. TB of kidney
D. Parathyroid adenoma

Let's discuss the options:

Option	*Statement*	*Remarks*
a	Ankylosing spondylitis	• Chronic back pain and progressive spinal stiffness is the usual presenting feature. • X-ray feature of early spondylitis is characterized by small erosions at the corners of vertebral bodies with reactive sclerosis: Romanus lesions of the spine (shiny corner sign). • Vertebral body squaring. • Non-infectious spondylodiscitis: Andersson lesion. • Diffuse syndesmophytic ankylosis can give a '**bamboo** spine' appearance. • Syndesmophytes are classically described as paravertebral ossification running parallel to the spine. • Linear ossification along the central spine; representing interspinous ligament ossification can give a '**dagger** spine' appearance on frontal radiographs of spine.

Contd.

b	Perforated peptic ulcer	• Patient presents with severe persistent pain in the epigastrium initially, later in the right side abdomen (as the inflammatory fluid spills along the right paracolic gutter) and finally become generalized. • Pain X-ray abdomen (erect posture) shows gas under diaphragm in 70% of cases.
c	TB of kidney	• Patient presents with frequency – both day and night. • Polyuria. • **Sterile pyuria:** Urine is pale and opalescent with presence of pus cells without organisms in an acid urine – bacterial aciduria. • Painful micturition with often hematuria. • Plain X-ray KUB – shows calcification.
d	Parathyroid adenoma	• Parathyroid adenomas are benign tumours of the parathyroid glands and are the **most** common cause of primary hyperparathyroidism. • Patient presents with elevated serum calcium levels and elevated serum parathyroid hormone levels. • This results in multisystem effects including osteoporosis, renal **calculi**, constipation, **peptic** ulcers, mental changes, **fatigue** and depression. • Clinical vignette of hyperparathyroidism – Bones, stones, abdominal groans and psychic moans. • X-ray skull show salt and **pepper** appearance. • Characteristic subperiosteal resorption may be seen on the radial aspect of the middle phalanges of the index and long fingers. • X-ray abdomen may show renal **stones**.

Coming back to the question:

- *A 30 years old male having abdominal pain (peptic ulcer), fatigue and dysuria (renal stone) might have parathyroid adenoma, which presents as hyperparathyroidism. X-ray abdomen might show renal stones.*

OBSTETRICS

1. Fetal heart rate accelerations are mediated by:

A. Chemoreceptor
B. Autonomic nervous system
C. Carotid baroreceptors
D. Aortic baroreceptors

Key points about accelerations in Fetal Heart Rate/FHR:

- *Transient increase in FHR by 15 beats per minute/bpm or more lasting for at least 15 seconds.*
- *Prolonged accelerations lasts $\geq$2 min but <10 min and when it is $\geq$10 min, it is a baseline change.*
- *Acceleration denotes an intact neurohormonal and cardiovascular activity and therefore a healthy fetus.*
- *FHR is controlled by the autonomic nervous system.*
- *The excitatory influence is conveyed by the* ***sympathetic*** *nervous system.*

Coming back to the question:

- *Fetal heart rate accelerations are mediated by autonomic nervous system.*

2. Which of the following transplacentally transmitted infection can cause probable anemia and myocarditis which can later develop into high output cardiac failure and ascites in fetus?

A. Cytomegalovirus
B. Toxoplasma gondii
C. Treponema pallidum
D. Parvovirus B19

Let's discuss the options:

Option	***Statement***	***Remarks***
a	Cytomegalovirus	• Fetus is affected by transplacental route in about 30-40% cases.

Contd.

		• Unlike rubella, CMV may damage fetal organs throughout gestation. • Amongst all infected foetuses only 10% will suffer serious damage. • The consequences of infection (5-18%) include miscarriage, non-immune hydrops, still birth, IUGR, microcephaly, intracranial calcification, hepatosplenomegaly, thrombocytopenia, choroidoretinitis, mental retardation and sensorineural deafness.
b	Toxoplasma gondii	• The fetal risk of infection **increases** with duration of pregnancy and is approximately 15%, 30% and 60% in the first, second and third trimesters respectively. • The fetus is **only** at risk if the mother is seronegative. • Risk of fetal damage **decreases** from 60% in first trimester to almost zero percent at the end of pregnancy. • There is increased rate of abortion, IUGR and stillbirth. • During parasitemia, transplacental infection to the foetuses occurs. • The affected baby may develop hydrocephalus, chorioretinitis, cerebral calcification, microcephaly, seizures and mental retardation.
c	Treponema pallidum	• Congenital infection results from transplacental migration of spirochete to the fetus. • Depending upon the intensity and time of occurrence of the infiltration, the fate of the fetus will be as follows: (1) Abortion (2) Preterm birth (3) Intrauterine deaths leading to either a macerated or a fresh stillbirth (4)

Contd.

		Non-immune fetal hydrops (ascites, hepatosplenomegaly) (5) Delivery of a highly infected baby with early neonatal death (6) Survival with congenital syphilis. • **Early** congenital syphilis: Maculopapular rash, rhinitis, hepatosplenomegaly, chorioretinitis. • **Late** congenital syphilis: Hutchinson teeth, deafness, saddle nose, saber shins, hydrocephalus, mental retardation, clutton joint, interstitial keratitis and optic nerve atrophy.
d	Parvovirus B19	• Parvovirus B19 (DNA) is associated with human infection (fifth disease) during pregnancy. • Fetal affection is by transplacental route. • Infection is characterized by facial rash (slapped cheek appearance). • It mainly affects the erythroid precursor cells resulting in **anemia**, thrombocytopenia, aplastic crises, congenital **heart failure** and **hydrops**. • Fetal injuries such as fetal **myocarditis**, endothelial lesions, and fetal cerebral damages have been reported. • Fetal loss is more when infection occurs early (<20 weeks) in pregnancy.

Coming back to the question:

- *Parvovirus is a transplacentally transmitted infection in fetus and can cause probable anemia, myocarditis which can later develop into high output cardiac failure and ascites.*

3. Non-immune hydrops fetalis is seen in all of the following EXCEPT:

A. Parvovirus B19 infection
B. Beta thalassemia
C. ABO incompatibility
D. Chromosomal abnormality

Key points about Nonimmune fetal hydrops/NIFH:

- *NIFH is defined as the accumulation of extracellular fluid in tissues and serous cavities in conditions other than Rh incompatibility.*
- *It is usually associated with increased skin thickness (> 5 mm), due to generalized subcutaneous edema in the fetus, placental enlargement, pericardial effusion, pleural effusion and/or ascites.*
- *With complete prevention of Rh problem, more than 75% of the fetal hydrops are related to NIFH.*
- *Causes of NIFH:*
    - o ***Chromosomal*** *abnormality (10%): Trisomies (13, 18, 21), Turner syndrome.*
    - o *Congenital cardiac lesions: Congenital heart block, supraventricular tachycardia.*
    - o *Congenital abnormalities: Diaphragmatic hernia, renal abnormality.*
    - o *Hematological: Beta-**thalassemia**, Glucose-6-Phosphate dehydrogenase deficiency.*
    - o *Infections: **Parvovirus**, rubella, toxoplasma, syphilis, cytomegalovirus.*
    - o *Placental and umbilical cord pathology: Twin-to-twin transfusion, chorioangioma.*
    - o *Maternal diseases: Uncontrolled diabetes, severe anemia.*

Coming back to the question:

- *ABO incompatibility leads to immune hydrops fetalis in fetus and not NIFH.*

4. All of the following maternal infections can be transmitted perinatally EXCEPT:

A. Herpes simplex virus
B. Hepatitis B
C. Rubella
D. Cytomegalovirus

Let's discuss the options:

Option	*Statement*	*Remarks*
a	Herpes simplex virus	• Transplacental infection is not usual. • The fetus becomes affected by virus shed from the cervix or lower genital tract during vaginal delivery. • The baby may be affected in utero from the contaminated liquor following rupture of the membranes.
b	Hepatitis B	• Perinatal transmission (10-40%) is high when viral load is high and presence of coinfection with HIV and HBV.
c	Rubella	• The virus predominantly affects the fetus and is extremely teratogenic if contracted within the **first** trimester. • Risk of major anomalies when this infection occurs in first, second and third month is approximately 60%, 25% and 10%, respectively.
d	Cytomegalovirus	• Fetus is affected by transplacental route in about 30-40% cases. • Virus is also excreted with urine, cervix and breast milk. • Unlike rubella, CMV may damage fetal organs throughout gestation.

Coming back to the question:

- *Rubella infection is not transmitted perinatally.*

GYNECOLOGY

1. A 28 weeks primigravida with fibroids presented to the ANC clinic with fever. Laboratory tests showed mild leucocytosis. Most likely diagnosis:

A. Secondary infection in fibroid
B. Red degeneration of fibroid
C. Torsion of fibroid
D. Sarcomatous change in fibroid

Let's discuss the options:

Option	*Statement*	*Remarks*
a	Secondary infection in fibroid	• The infection gains access to the tumour core through the thinned and sloughed surface epithelium of the submucous fibroid. • This usually happens following delivery or abortion. • Intramural fibroid may also be infected following delivery.
b	Red degeneration of fibroid	• Also known as carneous degeneration. • It occurs in a large fibroid mainly during second half of **pregnancy** and puerperium. • Partial recovery is possible and as such called necrobiosis. • The cause is not known but is probably vascular in origin. • Infection does **not** play any part. • Naked eye appearance of the tumour shows dark areas with cut section revealing raw-beef appearance often containing cystic spaces.

Contd.

		• The odour is often fishy due to fatty acids. • Color is due to the presence of hemolysed red cells and hemoglobin.
c	Torsion of fibroid	• Torsion of subserous pedunculated fibroid may lead to pain in lower abdomen.
d	Sarcomatous change in fibroid	• Sarcomatous change may occur in **less** than 0.1 percent cases. • The **usual** type is leiomyosarcoma. • Recurrence of fibroid polyp, sudden enlargement of fibroid or fibroid along with postmenopausal bleeding raises the **suspicion**.

Coming back to the question:

- *A pregnant lady in third trimester, with fibroids, might develop red degeneration of the fibroid.*

2. A 34 years' old multipara, with multiple sexual partners presented to the STD clinic with a painless vaginal ulcer. First investigation to be done in such a case is:

A. ELISA for HIV
B. Giemsa stain
C. VDRL
D. Scrapping from ulcer

Clinical presentation is indicative of primary syphilis.

Key points about syphilis:

- *It is caused by the anaerobic spirochete Treponema pallidum.*
- *Syphilitic lesion of the genital tract is acquired by direct contact with another person who has open primary or secondary syphilitic lesion.*
- *Transmission occurs through the abraded skin or mucosal surface.*
- *The incubation period ranges between 9 and 90 days.*
- *Primary lesion/chancre:*

- *May be a single or multiple and is usually located in the labia.*
- *Fourchette, anus, cervix and nipples are the other sites of lesion.*
- *A small papule is formed, which is quickly eroded to form an* ***ulcer****.*
- *The margins are raised with smooth shiny floor.*
- *The ulcer is* ***painless without*** *any surrounding inflammatory reaction.*
- *The inguinal glands are enlarged, discrete and painless.*
- *The primary chancre heals spontaneously in 1-8 weeks leaving behind a scar.*
- *The tubes are* ***not*** *affected and infertility does* ***not*** *occur.*

- *VDRL:*
  - *This is the* ***common*** *flocculation test performed and is positive after 6 weeks of initial infection.*
- *Specific tests:*
  - *Fluorescent treponemal antibody absorption test (FTA-abs) is expensive but a confirmatory test. FTA-IgM is produced only in active treponemal infection and it declines after adequate treatment.*
  - *Enzyme immunoassay/EIA test for treponemal specific IgG or IgM is now routinely used.*
  - *VDRL and TPHA tests are used for* ***screening*** *and FTA-abs test is used for* ***confirmation****.*

Coming back to the question:

- *Screening test (first investigation) in a suspected case of syphilis is VDRL.*

3. What is the reason for development of a female with complete gonadal dysgenesis and 46XY karyotype?

A. Mutation of SRY gene
B. Inversion of SRY gene
C. Deletion of SRY gene
D. Translocation of SRY gene

Key points about Swyer syndrome/Testicular Regression syndrome:

- *The individual presents with primary amenorrhoea.*
- *External genitalia are female.*

- *Internal genital organs are female.*
- *Secondary sexual characters are **absent**.*
- *Karyotype is 46, XY.*
- *Gonads are fibrous due to failure of development or regression.*
- *It is thought to be due to **mutation** in SRY gene at the Y chromosome.*
- *Gonadectomy is **recommended**.*
- *Estrogen and Progestin therapy is given for development of secondary sexual characters.*

Coming back to the question:

- *Development of a female with complete gonadal dysgenesis and 46XY karyotype is because of mutation of SRY gene.*

4. All of the following pairs (condition and surgical procedure) are correctly matched EXCEPT:

A. Uterovaginal prolapse – Hysterectomy with pelvic floor repair
B. Rectocele – Posterior colporrhaphy
C. Vault prolapse – Sacrospinous colpopexy
D. Cystourethrocele – Colposuspension

Let's discuss the options:

Option	***Statement***	***Remarks***
a	Uterovaginal prolapse	• Vaginal **hysterectomy** with pelvic floor repair/**PFR** is done. • The operation is often designated as Ward Mayo's operation named after Mayo (1915) and Ward (1919). • Removal of the uterus per vaginum (vaginal hysterectomy) is mostly done in cases of uterine prolapse. • It should be emphasized that hysterectomy is not the surgery for the prolapse. • It is the associated repair of the pelvic floor/PFR, which is the corrective surgery for prolapse.

Contd.

b	Rectocele	• Rectocele is defined as a defect in the rectovaginal septum, causing symptoms like obstructed defecation syndrome (ODS), vaginal bulging etc. • Once the rectocele is larger than 3 cm and/or symptomatic, surgery should be considered. • The surgical approach can be either transvaginal, transanal or transperineal. • Two of the most common procedures in treating rectocele are **posterior** colporrhaphy (PC) and stapled trans-anal rectal resection (STARR).
c	Vault prolapse	• Post-hysterectomy (vaginal or abdominal) vault prolapse is usually accompanied by an enterocele (70%). • The vault prolapse in such cases may be effectively repaired transvaginally maintaining the same principle of repair of enterocele along with anterior colporrhaphy and colpoperineorrhaphy. • Sometimes, it may require suspension of the vault with the anterior sacral ligament in front of 3rd sacral vertebra (sacrospinous **colpopexy**) transabdominally using non-absorbable sutures such as Teflon or Mersilene mesh. • The sacrospinous ligament is attached medially to the sacrum and coccyx and laterally to the ischial spine. • Vaginal vault is fixed to the coccygenus sacrospinous ligament complex (CSSL) of the right side.
d	Cysto-urethrocele	• **Anterior** colporrhaphy is designed to correct cystocele and urethrocele.

Contd.

		• The underlying principles are to excise a portion of the relaxed anterior vaginal wall, to mobilize the bladder and push it upwards after cutting the vesicocervical ligament. • The bladder is then permanently supported by plicating the endopelvic fascia and the pubocervical fascia under the bladder neck in the midline.

Coming back to the question:

- *Colposuspension/Retropubic cystourethropexy is done in genuine stress incontinence/GSI.*

5. True statements regarding primary dysmenorrhoea are all EXCEPT:

A. Psychological factor is involved
B. GnRH analogue is the first line of management
C. Seen only in adolescent girls
D. Pain starts 24 hours prior to the menses and resolves by 2 days

Key points about Primary dysmenorrhoea/Spasmodic:

- *Dysmenorrhoea literally means painful menstruation.*
- *The primary dysmenorrhoea is one where there is **no** identifiable pelvic pathology.*
- *Mostly confined to **adolescents**.*
- *Pain is always confined to the ovulatory cycles.*
- *The pain is usually cured following pregnancy and vaginal delivery.*
- *The pain is related to dysrhythmic uterine contractions and uterine hypoxia.*
- ***Psychosomatic** factors of tension and anxiety during adolescence is one important factor for pain; lower the pain threshold.*
- *The pain begins a few hours **before** or just with the onset of menstruation.*
- *The severity of pain usually **lasts** for few hours, may extend to 24 hours but seldom persists beyond 48 hours.*

- *The pain is spasmodic and confined to lower abdomen; may radiate to the back and medial aspects of thighs.*
- *Abdominal or pelvic examination does **not** reveal any abnormal findings.*
- *The drugs used in management are:*
    - o ***PSI**/Prostaglandin synthetase inhibitors: These drugs not only reduce the prostaglandin synthesis (by inhibition of cyclo-oxygenase enzyme) but also have a direct analgesic effect. These drugs can be used orally for 2-3 days starting with the onset of period. The drug should be continued for 3-6 cycles.*
    - o ***OCP**/Oral contraceptives are prescribed to patients, in whom PSI are contraindicated or patients who want contraception too.*

Coming back to the question:

- *PSI (Mefenamic acid/Ibuprofen/Indomethacin) are used in managing primary dysmenorrhoea (not GnRH analogues).*

6. A patient of bacterial vaginosis presented with grey white discharge. Clue cells were seen. Which of the following statement define clue cells?

A. Vaginal epithelial cells covered with bacilli
B. Neutrophils
C. Chain of Gardnerella vaginalis
D. Macrophages with Doderlein bacilli

Key points about Clue cells:

- *A smear of vaginal discharge is prepared with drops of normal saline on a glass slide and is seen under a microscope.*
- *Vaginal epithelial cells are seen covered with these coccobacilli and the cells appear as stippled or granular.*
- *At times, the cells are so heavily stippled that the cell borders are obscured.*
- *These stippled epithelial cells are called 'clue cells'.*
- *Presence of clue cells (>20% of cells) are **diagnostic** of bacterial vaginosis.*

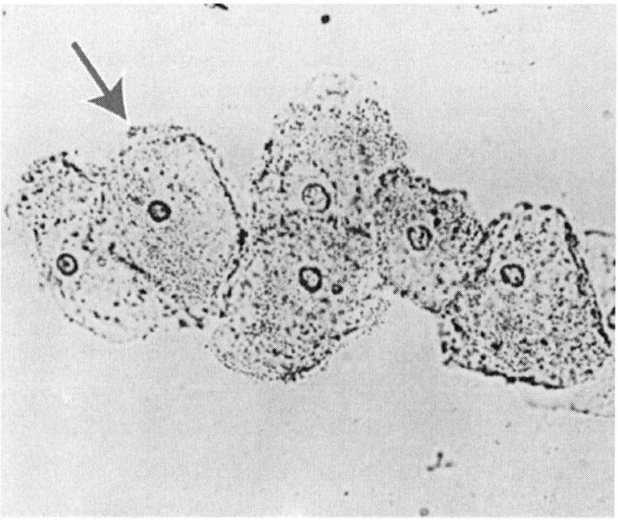

Coming back to the question:

- *Clue cells are epithelial cells of the vagina that get their distinctive stippled appearance by being covered with bacteria.*

7. A known case of dyspareunia and dysmenorrhoea presented to the fertility clinic. On abdominal examination a mass was felt, which was tender with restricted mobility. Uterus was fixed and retroverted. Hysterosalpingography showed spill on both the sides. Such a case is best investigated by:

A. Transvaginal Sonography/TVS
B. Biopsy
C. MRI
D. Laparoscopy

Clinical presentation is indicative of endometriosis.

Let's discuss the options:

Option	*Statement*	*Remarks*
a	Transvaginal USG	• USG is **not** much helpful to the diagnosis. • TVS can detect ovarian endometriomas. • TVS and Endorectal ultrasound are found **better** for rectosigmoid endometriosis.

Contd.

b	Biopsy	• Biopsy confirmation of excised lesion is **ideal** but negative histology does not exclude endometriosis.
c	MRI	• Magnetic Resonance Imaging is a **diagnostic** tool. • There is characteristic hyperintensity on T1 weighted images and a hypointensity on T2 weighted images.
d	Laparoscopy	• Laparoscopy is the **gold** standard. • It can confirm the lesion with site, size and extent. • Biopsy can be taken at the same time. • Staging can be done. • Extent of adhesions could be recorded. • Opportunity to do laparoscopic surgery, if needed. • The **classic** lesion of pelvic endometriosis is described as 'powder burns' or 'match stick' spots on the peritoneum of the pouch of Douglas.

Coming back to the question:

- *Laparoscopy is the gold standard investigation for endometriosis.*

8. A male presented with azoospermia, acidic semen with absent fructose. On evaluation, FSH and LH levels were found to be normal. Most likely diagnosis:

A. Hypothalamic failure
B. Pituitary failure
C. Testicular atrophy
D. Obstruction of vas deferens

Key points about Evaluation of a patient with azoospermia/ Oligospermia:

- *Azoospermia means no spermatozoan in the semen.*
- *Oligospermia/Oligozoospermia means sperm count is less than 20 million per mL.*

- *Fructose content in the seminal fluid:*
  - o *Its **absence** suggests congenital absence of seminal vesicle or partial duct obstruction or both.*
- *Serum FSH, LH, testosterone (TST), prolactin (PL) and TSH:*
  - o *Testicular dysfunction causes rise in FSH and LH.*
  - o *Low level of FSH and LH suggest hypogonadotropic hypogonadism.*
  - o *Leydig cell dysfunction causes low TST and high LH level.*
  - o *Elevated PL due to pituitary adenoma may cause impotency.*
- *Testicular biopsy:*
  - o *It is done to differentiate primary testicular failure from obstruction as a cause of azoospermia or severe oligospermia.*
  - o *The biopsy material is to be sent in Bouin's solution and **not** in formal saline.*

Coming back to the question:

- *Absent fructose in seminal fluid with normal FSH and LH level suggest obstruction of vas deferens, as a cause of azoospermia.*

9. Which of the following are true statements for primary amenorrhoea?

I. Raised TSH with short stature
II. No menarche by 16 years
III. No thelarche and menarche by 14 years
IV. Gap of more than 3 years between menarche and thelarche

Lead – Choose the best answer from the codes given below:

A. I and II B. II and III
C. I, II and III D. I, II, III and IV

Let's discuss the options:

Option	***Statement***	***Remarks***
I	Raised TSH with short stature	• False statement. • Raised TSH suggest hypothyroidism.

Contd.

		• Hypothyroidism can also slow down the growth rate of height. • Hypothyroidism causes secondary amenorrhoea.
II	No menarche by 16 years	• True statement. • A young girl who has **not** yet menstruated by her 16 years of age is having primary amenorrhoea rather than delayed menarche. • The **normal** upper age limit for menarche is 15 years.
III	No thelarche and menarche by 14 years	• True statement. • Females who have **not** reached menarche at 14 years and who have **no** signs of secondary sexual characteristics (thelarche or pubarche) are also considered to have primary amenorrhoea.
IV	Gap of more than 3 years between menarche and thelarche	• False statement. • As obvious from above points, gap between thelarche and menarche is 2 years (14 years and 16 years).

Coming back to the question:

- *A girl who has no menstrual period by the age of 14 years (in the absence of secondary sexual characters) or by the age of 16 years (in the presence of normal secondary sexual characters) is having primary amenorrhoea.*

10. All of the following are effects of HRT/hormone replacement therapy EXCEPT:

A. High risk of breast cancer
B. High risk of colon cancer
C. Low risk of hip fracture
D. High risk of endometrial cancer

Let's discuss the options:

Option	*Statement*	*Remarks*
a	High risk of breast cancer	• True statement. • Combined estrogen and progestin replacement therapy, **increases** the risk of breast cancer lightly (RR 1.26). • Adverse effects of HRT are related to the dose and duration of the therapy.
b	High risk of colon cancer	• False statement. • HRT **reduces** chances of colo-rectal cancer (20%).
c	Low risk of hip fracture	• True statement. • HRT prevents bone loss and stimulate new bone formation. • HRT increases bone mineral density/BMD by 2-5% and **reduces** the risk of vertebral and hip fracture (25-50%). • Estrogen is found to play a direct role, as receptors have been found in the osteoclasts.
d	High risk of endometrial cancer	• True statement. • When estrogen is given alone to a woman with intact uterus, it causes endometrial proliferation, hyperplasia and carcinoma. • It is therefore advised that a progestogen should be added to estrogen/ERT to counter balance such risks.

Coming back to the question:

- *HRT causes reduction in colorectal cancer by 20%.*

11. Which of the following is the most common cause of pubertal menorrhagia?

A. Endometriosis
B. Bleeding diathesis
C. Malignancy
D. Anovulatory cycles

Key points about Abnormal Uterine Bleeding/AUB:

- *AUB is the **most** common gynecologic complaint of adolescents admitted to the hospital.*
- *Heavy menstrual bleeding/HMB is the **most** frequent clinical presentation of AUB.*
- ***Anovulatory** cycles, owing to immature hypothalamic-pituitary-ovarian axis, is the **leading** etiology of HMB and there is an accompanying bleeding disorder in almost 20% of the patients with HMB.*
    - o *Anovular bleeding is usually excessive.*
    - o *In the absence of growth limiting progesterone due to anovulation, the endometrial growth is under the influence of estrogen throughout the cycle.*
    - o *There is inadequate structural stromal support and the endometrium remains fragile.*
    - o *Thus, with the withdrawal of estrogen due to negative feedback action of FSH, the endometrial shedding continues for a longer period in asynchronous sequences because of lack of compactness.*
- *Additionally, endocrine disorders such as hypothyroidism, hyper-prolactinemia and polycystic ovary syndrome are possible causes of AUB.*
- *Exclusion of bleeding disorders, especially von Willebrand disease is important for diagnosis and treatment of HMB, particularly in cases with AUB, which has been present since menarche.*

Coming back to the question:

- *Anovulatory cycle is the most common cause of pubertal menorrhagia.*

12. A female presented with infertility since 6 years. She is having hirsutism. Her body mass index is 30. USG showed polycystic ovaries. What will be best advice for such a case?

A. Finasteride + Ovulation induction agents
B. Finasteride + Metformin
C. Weight loss + Metformin + Urinary gonadotropin
D. Weight loss + Metformin + Clomiphene citrate

Key points about management of PCOS/Polycystic Ovarian Syndrome:

- *Weight reduction:*
  - *Weight reduction in obese patients is the first line of treatment.*
  - *Body Mass Index (BMI) <25 improves menstrual disorders, infertility, impaired glucose intolerance (insulin resistance), hyperandrogenemia (hirsutism, acne) and obesity.*
  - *Weight **reduction** (2-5%) improves the metabolic syndrome and reproductive function.*
- *Ovulation induction:*
  - *It is usually achieved by **Clomiphene** citrate following correction of other biochemical abnormalities.*
  - *In unresponsive cases, pure FSH or HMG along with hCG may be administered with monitoring facilities.*
- *Insulin sensitizers:*
  - *Women with PCOS and hyperinsulinemia with BMI >25, ovulate satisfactorily when Clomiphene is combined with metformin.*
  - ***Metformin** improves metabolic syndrome by reducing all the parameters: weight, BMI (hyperinsulinemia, hyperandrogenism), blood pressure and lipid abnormalities.*
  - *500 mg thrice daily is found to correct the biochemical abnormalities.*
  - *Pioglitazone and Rosiglitazone are also being used in cases, resistant to metformin.*

Coming back to the question:

- *Weight loss + Metformin + Clomiphene citrate is useful in a PCOS patient desirous of pregnancy.*

13. All of the following are used in managing endometriosis EXCEPT:

A. Leuprolide B. Danazol
C. Estrogen valerate D. Medroxyprogesterone

Key points about Hormonal treatment of Endometriosis:

- *The **aim** of the hormonal treatment is to induce atrophy of the endometriotic implants.*
- *It should be considered suppressive rather than curative because of **high** recurrence rate.*
- *The mechanism of endometrial atrophy is either by producing 'pseudopregnancy' (Combined oral pills) or by 'pseudomenopause' (Danazol) or by 'Medical oophorectomy' (GnRH agonists).*
- *All the drugs are used continuously to produce amenorrhoea.*
- *The hormonal use is gratifying in superficial peritoneal implants and endometriosis of less than 1 cm.*
- *For **quick** relief of symptoms and reduction of the volume of the lesion, GnRH analogues are the best.*
- *Progestogens take some time to achieve these objectives.*
- *Danazol is placed midway between the two.*
- *Taking every aspect together (pain relief, pregnancy rates, recurrence rates, costs and side-effects), **no** single medical treatment is superior to others.*
- *Combined estrogen and progestogen:*
  - *The low dose contraceptive pills may be prescribed either in a cyclic or continuous fashion with advantages in young patients with mild disease who want to defer pregnancy.*
  - *It causes endometrial decidualization and atrophy.*
  - *It may induce amenorrhoea.*
  - *It relieves dysmenorrhoea.*
- *Progestogens:*
  - *It causes decidualization of endometrium and atrophy.*
  - *High doses may suppress ovulation and induce amenorrhoea.*
  - *Oral route is commonly used.*
  - *Orally used agents are **Medroxyprogesterone** acetate/ Dydrogesterone/Norethisterone*

- *Danazol:*
  - o ***Danazol** therapy is to be started from the day 5 of the menstrual cycle.*
  - o *The dose (600-800 mg daily) is variable and depends upon the extent of the lesions but should be adequate enough to produce amenorrhoea.*
  - o *The patient should use barrier methods of contraception to avoid virilisation of a female fetus in accidental pregnancy.*
  - o *Resolution of endometriotic lesions has been seen in about 80% of cases but the recurrence rate is high (40%).*
- *GnRH analogues:*
  - o *When used continuously, act as medical oophorectomy, a state of hypoestrinism and amenorrhoea.*
  - o *The goal is to maintain a **low** level of serum estrogen (30-45 pg/mL) so that growth of endometriosis is suppressed.*
  - o *The side effects are more tolerable than Danazol.*
  - o *Members in this group are **Leuprolide**, Naferelin and Goserelin*

Coming back to the question:

- *Estrogen valerate is not used in the management of endometriosis.*

14. All of the following tests are significant in Turner syndrome EXCEPT:

A. Audiometry
B. Echocardiography
C. Glucose tolerance test
D. Anti-nuclear antibody

Key points about evaluation of Turner syndrome/TS:

- *Cardiac evaluation:*
  - o *A congenital heart defect (CHD) occurs in approximately 30% of patients with TS.*
  - o *Of those with a CHD, left-sided obstructive defects **predominate**, especially bicuspid aortic valve (BAV; 30-50%) and coarctation of aorta (COA; 30%).*
  - o *At the time of diagnosis, all individuals, regardless of age, should have a cardiac evaluation including a complete physical examination and an **echocardiogram**.*

- *Evaluation of renal anatomy:*
  - o *Congenital malformations of the urinary system are present in up to 30% of the patients with TS.*
  - o *Rotational abnormalities and double collecting systems are found* ***most*** *frequently.*
  - o *Therefore, all individuals with TS should have a renal ultrasound study performed at the time of diagnosis.*
- *Blood pressure:*
  - o *Hypertension is* ***common*** *in TS, even in the absence of cardiac of renal malformations.*
  - o *Blood pressure should therefore be monitored at each physical examination.*
- *Thyroid function:*
  - o *Between 10 and 30% of individuals with TS develop primary hypothyroidism, generally associated with anti-thyroid anti-bodies.*
  - o *Level of TSH and total or free T4 should therefore be measured at the time of diagnosis and at intervals of 1-2 year thereafter.*
- *Hearing:*
  - o *Conductive and sensorineural hearing loss are* ***common*** *in girls with TS.*
  - o *The outer, middle and inner ear are all affected, and hearing problems and ear malformations correlate with the karyotype.*
  - o ***Audiometry*** *must be carried out.*
- *Vision:*
  - o *Strabismus, amblyopia and ptosis are* ***common*** *in TS.*
  - o *Ophthalmological evaluation should be a part of the regular physical examination.*
- *Orthopedic evaluation:*
  - o *Infants with TS have an increased* ***risk*** *of congenital hip dislocation, which may be associated with degenerative arthritis of the hips in older women.*
  - o *Orthopedic evaluation must be done.*

- *Glucose intolerance:*
    - o *Although there may be an increased **risk** of glucose tolerance, frank diabetes is **rare** in children with TS.*
    - o *Routine **glucose** tolerance tests can be done.*

Coming back to the question:

- *Anti-nuclear antibody detection (ANA) is not a part of evaluation of Turner syndrome.*

15. A female patient, who was on oral contraceptive pills, presented with white vaginal discharge, staining undergarments yellow. There was no soreness or itching. pH of vagina was acidic. Microscopy showed large number of normal lactobacilli. Most likely diagnosis:

A. Candidiasis
B. Bacterial vaginosis
C. Trichomoniasis
D. Physiological

Let's discuss the options:

Option	*Statement*	*Remarks*
a	Candidiasis	• Also known as candida vaginitis/ moniliasis. • **Predisposing factors:** Diabetes, pregnancy, broad spectrum antibiotics, OCPs, HIV, steroids etc. • Patient complains of vaginal discharge with intense vulvovaginal **pruritus**. • The pruritus is **out** of proportion to the discharge. • The discharge is thick, curdy white and in flakes (**cottage** cheese type) often adherent to the vaginal wall. • Vulva may be **red** and swollen with evidences of pruritus. • Vaginal examination may be tender.

Contd.

		• Removal of the white flakes reveals multiple oozing points. • Wet smear of vaginal discharge (with KOH solution) shows filamentous forms of mycelia, pseudo-hyphae (under microscope).
b	Bacterial vaginosis	• BV is characterised clinically by creamy vaginal discharge with fishy smell without extensive evidence of **inflammation**. • The discharge is homogenous, greyish-white and adherent to the vaginal wall. • **Amsel's four diagnostic criteria:** (1) Homogenous vagina discharge (2) Vaginal **pH** >4.5 (3) Positive Whiff test (4) Presence of clue cells (>20%). • Gram stained vaginal smear (Hay/Ison): Presence of more Gardnerella or mobiluncus morphotypes with few or **absent** lactobacilli.
c	Trichomoniasis	• **Predisposing conditions:** When the local defence is impaired – during and after menstruation, after sexual stimulation, and following illness, the **pH** of the vagina is raised to 5.5 – 6.5. • There is sudden profuse and offensive vaginal discharge often dating from the last menstruation. • The discharge is thin, greenish-yellow and frothy offensive. • Irritation and itching of varying degrees within and around the introits are **common**. • The vulva is inflamed with evidence of **pruritus**. • The vaginal walls become **red** and inflamed with multiple punctate hemorrhagic spots.

Contd.

		• Similar spots are also found over the mucosa of the portio vaginalis part of the cervix on speculum examination giving the appearance of '**strawberry**'. • There is presence of urinary symptoms such as dysuria and frequency of micturition. • Identification of the trichomonas is done by hanging drop preparation.
d	Physiological	• Leucorrhea can be seen with **OCPs** use. • It may be due to excessive cervical mucus secretion (estrogen) or due to increased preponderance of monilial infection (estrogen + progestin).

Coming back to the question:

- *Female patient, on oral contraceptive pills, presenting with white vaginal discharge (staining undergarments yellow) without any soreness or itching, with acidic vaginal pH and microscopy showing large number of normal lactobacilli suggest the development of leucorrhoea (an adverse effect of OCPs).*

16. A female at puberty, presents with primary amenorrhoea. The karyotype was 46 XY. Breast development was adequate but vagina was short and blind. Clitoromegaly was noted. Axillary and pubic hairs were absent. Testosterone level was normal. Most likely diagnosis:

A. Androgen insensitivity syndrome
B. 17-hydroxylase deficiency
C. Swyer syndrome
D. 5-alpha reductase type 2 deficiency

Let's discuss the options:

Option	***Statement***	***Remarks***
a	Androgen insensitivity syndrome	• Also known as testicular feminization.

Contd.

		• The underlying pathology is the **inability** of the endorgans to respond to androgens. • Either there is lack of androgen cytosol receptor or the receptor is defective (mutated). • They are phenotypically and psychologically **female**. • Usually presents with primary **amenorrhoea** and/or infertility. • **Breast** development is adequate. • Nipples are small with pale areola. • There is eunuchoidal tendency (long arms, big hands and feets). • **Absent** or sparse axillary and pubic hairs. • External genitalia look female. • **Clitoris** is enlarged. • **Vagina** is short and blind. • The upper two-thirds of vagina, uterus and tubes are **absent** due to the effect of AMH (anti-Mullerian Hormone). • The gonads (Sertoli cell) secrete AMH. • Gonads (testes) are either placed in the labia, or inguinal canal or intra-abdominal. • Karyotype is **46, XY**. • Serum **testosterone** is within average for normal males.
b	17-hydroxylase deficiency	• Steroid 17-hydroxylase is a cytochrome p450 enzyme.

Contd.

		• It hydroxylates pregnenolone and progesterone (which are precursors to aldosterone) to form 17-OH pregnenolone and 17-OH progesterone (which are precursors to cortisol). • 17-OH pregnenolone and 17-OH progesterone are also precursors to DHEA and androstenedione, respectively. • Patients with a 17hydroxylase deficiency **cannot** synthesize cortisol or sex hormones effectively. • The deficiency in cortisol production results in disruption of the feedback loop to the hypothalamic-pituitary axis and a resultant overproduction of ACTH, which in turn leads to hyperplasia of the adrenal cortex. • The inability to effectively synthesize sex hormones results in a range of defect in sexual maturation. • There is resultant excess on 11-deoxycorticosterone and corticosterone. • Aldosterone levels may vary and can range from low to high. • Patients with 17-hydroxylase deficiency may present with hypertension and hypokalemia in childhood or adulthood due to the mineralocorticoid **excess** that develops in the presence of excess ACTH. • The additional presenting features will differ based on genotypic sex and are associated with deficient sex hormone production, which will typically **not** manifest until puberty. • **46, XX**: Female patient do not develop hypertension or hypokalemia before puberty.

Contd.

		• They will generally present with complaints of delayed puberty, primary amenorrhea, and **lack** of secondary sexual characteristics. • **46, XY:** Presentation can range from phenotypic females to ambiguous or small male genitalia. • They also present with complaints of delayed puberty, primary amenorrhea, and **lack** of secondary sexual characteristics. • On physical examination, they will have a blind pouch instead of a vagina and lack internal female genitalia. • The testes are undescended or located in the inguinal canal.
c	Swyer syndrome	• Also known as testicular regression syndrome. • The individual presents with primary amenorrhoea. • External genitalia are female. • Internal organs are female. • Secondary sexual characters are **absent**. • Karyotype is 46, XY. • Gonads are fibrous due to failure of development or regression. • It is thought to be mutation in SRY gene at the Y chromosome.
d	5-alpha reductase type 2 deficiency	• The 5α-RD2 enzyme converts testosterone/TST into a more potent form of the male sex hormone called DHT (dihydrotestosterone). • During male fetal development, TST and DHT have a specific predetermined role in sexual development.

Contd.

		• TST is the driver for the development of male internal genitalia, including the Wolffian duct, whereas DHT has a role in the genesis of male external genitalia. • At puberty, TST is responsible for aggressive psychosexual behaviour, deepening of the voice, increased muscle mass, and initiating spermatogenesis. • Children with deficiency of 5α-reductase will have **decreased** production of DHT during fetal development, and this leads to defective external genital development and ambiguous genitalia. • 5alpha-RD2 deficiency is one of the **important** causes of ambiguous genitalia in children. • The phenotype of children with 5α-RD2 deficiency can vary from underdeveloped male genitalia to a complete female phenotype. • The genotype of these children is 46 XY. • The newborns might have genitalia resembling labia majora, which in reality would be unfused labioscrotal folds. • The phallus in these children may look more like a clitoris than a penis. • At the same time, the internal genitalia in these children will include seminal vesicles, epididymis, vas deferens, and ejaculatory duct, and one may **not** see any Mullerian structures.

Contd.

		• The testes in these children might be present in the inguinal sac, and very rarely, they can also be found within the abdomen. • These children tend to be raised as females till puberty, by which time they start exhibiting virilisation. • At puberty, the phallus may grossly enlarge to forma a penis, the testes may descend into the unfused labioscrotal folds, the voice deepens, and a beard starts growing. • The development of all these secondary sexual characteristics during puberty does **not** need the presence of DHT but **only** the presence of TST.

Coming back to the question:

- *A female having primary amenorrhoea with 46, XY karyotype, adequate breast development, short and blind vagina, clitoromegaly, absent axillary and pubic hairs and a normal testosterone level suggest the possibility of androgen insensitivity syndrome.*

DERMATOLOGY

1. Which of the following is a specific antibody for dermatomyositis?

A. Anti-nuclear antibody
B. Anti-centromere antibody
C. Anti-Mi-2 antibody
D. Anti-Smith antibody

Let's discuss the options:

Option	*Statement*	*Remarks*
a	Anti-nuclear antibody	• ANAs are a class of antibodies that bind to cellular components in the nucleus, including proteins, DNA, RNA and nucleic acid-protein complexes. • ANAs are possible signs of autoimmune diseases, such as lupus, scleroderma, Sjogren's syndrome, juvenile arthritis, or polymyositis and dermatomyositis.
b	Anti-centromere antibody	• ACAs are detected in patients with various autoimmune diseases such as Sjogren's syndrome (SS), systemic sclerosis (SSc) and primary biliary cirrhosis (PBC).
c	Anti-Mi-2 antibody	• The anti-Mi-2 antibody is a **dermatomyositis** (DM)-specific autoantibody.
d	Anti-Smith antibody	• Anti-Smith (Sm) antibody is a **highly** specific antibody for systemic lupus erythematosus (SLE).

Coming back to the question:

- *Anti-Mi-2 antibody is highly specific for classic dermatomyositis.*

2. Identify the lines shown in the image:

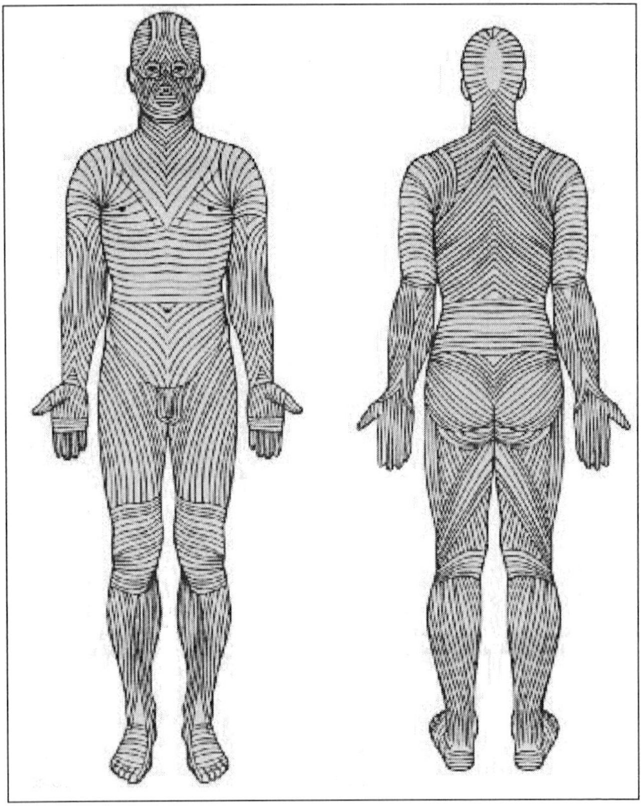

A. Blaschko lines

B. Relaxed skin tension lines

C. Marionettes lines

D. Wrinkle lines

Let's discuss the options:

Option	*Statement*	*Remarks*
a	Blaschko lines	• It refers to a system of lines representing the developmental growth pattern of human skin **irrespective** of any known nervous, vascular or lymphatic structures. • Many linear nevi and dermatosis follow these lines.

Contd.

b	Relaxed skin tension lines	• RSTL are **imaginary** lines along which maximal forces are generated by the skin in conjunction with underlying muscle, collagen fibers and fibrous bands. • RSTL are produced in living subjects by positioning the body so that the skin is relaxed, and then gently pinching the skin to reveal a creases.
c	Marionettes lines	• Marionette lines are facial wrinkles that occur with natural aging. • The lines run vertically between the mouth and chin, which can create sagging in the lower half of the face.
d	Wrinkle lines	• Wrinkle lines were described by Kraissl and were based on photographs of an elderly man with wrinkles. • Wrinkle line do **not** always align with tension lines, particularly on the chin, dorsum of the nose, and the area lateral to the eyes.

Coming back to the question:

- *RSTL refer to furrows that are created when the skin is pinched and relaxed.*

3. A 55 years old male is on Nivolumab. He had pruritic and urticarial lesion. Histopathological examination showed subepidemral cleft. Direct immunofluorescence/DIF showed linear deposits of IgG and C3 along the dermoepidermal junction. Most likely diagnosis:

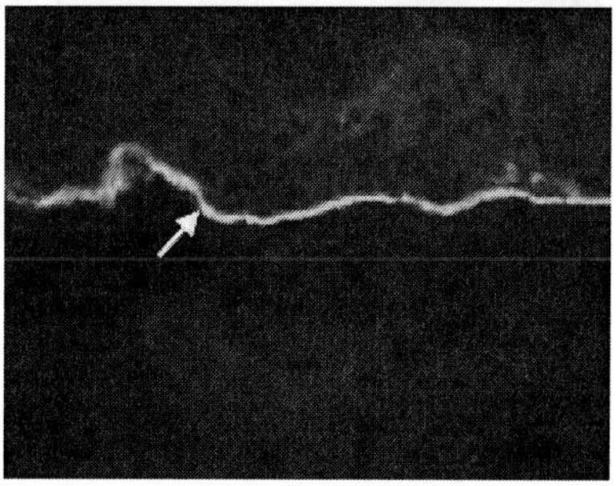

A. Pemphigus vulgaris
B. Bullous pemphigoid
C. Dermatitis herpetiformis
D. Pemphigus foliaceus

Let's discuss the options:

Option	*Statement*	*Remarks*
a	Pemphigus vulgaris	• Pemphigus is an autoimmune disease, which is characterized by intraepidermal blistering at various levels in the epidermis, because of disruption of the intercellular cementing substance. • It is due to an autoantibody attack (IgG) on the cellular adhesion proteins (desmogliens/ DG) leading to acantholysis seen on Tzanck smear. • Antibody: IgG1 and C3 against DG3. • **Drugs:** Sulfydryl group-penicillamine, Captopril, Rifampicin etc. • Mucosal lesions are seen in **all** the patients. • Either the onset is with painful oral erosions (50-70%) or is involved during the course of the disease. • Skin lesions are asymptomatic, flaccid bullae on normal or erythematous skin. • **Histopathological** examination shows a **suprabasal** cleft in the epidermis containing eosinophils and acantholytic cells. • The basal keratinocytes remain attached to the basement membrane but are separated from each other and stand like a 'row of tombstones'. • **DIF** from the lesional skin will have deposition of intercellular IgG throughout the epidermis in a 'fish-net' pattern (IgG, IgA, C3, C1q).

Contd.

b	Bullous pemphigoid	• Bullous pemphigoid is an autoimmune skin disorder characterized by subepidermal blistering which results in large, tense bullae. • Pathogenesis include formation of IgG antibodies against components of the basement membrane zone (BMZ – structure which binds epidermis to the underlying dermis and mesenchyme). • This leads to loss of structural integrity of the BMZ due to resultant inflammation and separation of the intact epidermis from underlying dermis and forms a **subepidermal** cleft containing eosinophils and neutrophils. • **Antigen:** Hemidesmosome (BPAg1 and BPAg2). • **Drugs implicated:** Benzodiazepine, Furosemide, Penicillin, Sulfasalazine, **Novilumab**. • Lesion starts as **urticarial** wheals, which are preceded by **itching**. • It lasts for 1-3 weeks and finally dense bullae on normal or erythematous skin predominantly over flexural aspects of the limbs, lower abdomen, groins and axillae are formed. • **DIF:** Linear **IgG** (45-90%) and **C3** (80-100%) deposition in BMZ.
c	Dermatitis herpetiformis	• DH is an intensely pruritic, chronic skin disease characterized by papulovesicular lesions and urticarial wheals located on the extensor surfaces in a symmetric distribution. • The disease persists indefinitely, and is associated with a gluten-sensitive enteropathy in most patients.

Contd.

		• IgA antibody against Gliadin cross reacts to the intestinal epithelium and that reacts with an antigen in the skin TGII. • The lesions of DH usually begin as a vesicle, but may also be erythematous papules, urticarial like wheals, excoriations, crusts, or rarely, large bullae. • The lesions are usually intensely pruritic, accompanied by burning and stinging. • **Histopathological** examination shows neutrophilic microabscesses in the dermal papillae, dermal infiltration of neutrophils and eosinophils, and the formation of **subepidermal** vesicles. • **DIF** reveals granular deposition of **IgA** in the tips of dermal papillae. • In areas corresponding to IgA deposits, there may also be complement deposition.
d	Pemphigus foliaceus	• It is less severe than pemphigus vulgaris and is characterized by crusted, moist, scaly lesions in a seborrheic distribution involving scalp, face, chest and upper back. • Bullous lesions may **not** be seen because of the superficial level of the split that may cause erosions, scaling and crusting. • Oral lesions are **absent**. • Antibody is IgG and is against DG1 (Desmoglein 1). • The acantholytic cell is cuboidal in shape.

Coming back to the question:

- *Bullous pemphigoid can be seen after Nivolumab therapy, and the patient presents with pruritic and urticarial lesions. Histopathological examination shows subepidermal cleft. Direct immunofluorescence/DIF shows linear deposits of IgG and C3 along the dermoepidermal junction.*

4. Match the following:

Condition	***Woods lamp appearance***
1. Pityriasis versicolor	**A. Green**
2. Vitiligo	**B. White**
3. Tinea capitis	**C. Yellow**
4. Erythrasma	**D. Coral red**

Lead – Choose the best answer from the codes given below:

A. 1-B, 2-A, 3-D, 4-C
B. 1-C, 2-B, 3-A, 4-D
C. 1-A, 2-B, 3-C, 4-D
D. 1-C, 2-A, 3-B, 4-D

Let's discuss the options:

Option	***Statement***	***Remarks***
1	Pityriasis versicolor	• The previous name tinea versicolor is no longer used. • It is a mild chronic opportunistic infection of skin caused by yeast Malasezzia. • It is asymptomatic. • Pruritus is **not** a feature. • **Wood's lamp examination:** Lesions may show pale or golden **yellow** fluorescence.
2	Vitiligo	• It is an acquired idiopathic hypomelanotic disorder which presents as localized or widespread areas of depigmentation. • **Wood's lamp examination:** Lesions appear more **white**.

Contd.

3	Tinea capitis	• It includes infection of both scalp and hair. • It is predominantly seen in children (3-14 years). • But it is **uncommon** in adults. • **Wood's lamp examination:** Ectothrix type of tinea capitis caused by Microsporum audouinii and M. canis produced yellow-**green** fluorescence.
4	Erythrasma	• It is an asymptomatic, irregularly shaped, sharply marginated red or brown patches in axillae, groins and submammary and intergluteal regions. • **Wood's lamp examination:** Erythrasma caused by Corynebacterium minutissimum produces a porphyrin compound which fluoresces a bright red color (**coral** red).

Coming back to the question:

Condition	***Woods lamp appearance***
1. Pityriasis versicolor	*C. Yellow*
2. Vitiligo	*B. White*
3. Tinea capitis	*A. Green*
4. Erythrasma	*D. Coral red*

5. Read the following statements:

Assertion: Histological examination of a patient with flaccid bullae shows suprabasal splitting

Reason: Row of tombstones is seen in pemphigus vulgaris and is diagnostic

A. Both are true but reason is the correct explanation of assertion
B. Both are true but reason is not the correct explanation of assertion
C. Assertion is true but reason is false
D. Assertion is false but reason is true

Key points about Histology of Pemphigus vulgaris:

- *Histopathological examination shows a **suprabasal** cleft in the epidermis containing eosinophils and acantholytic cells.*
- *Suprabasal cell shows loss of intercellular adhesions (acantholysis).*
- *The basal keratinocytes remain attached to the basement membrane but are separated from each other and stand like a '**row** of tombstones'.*

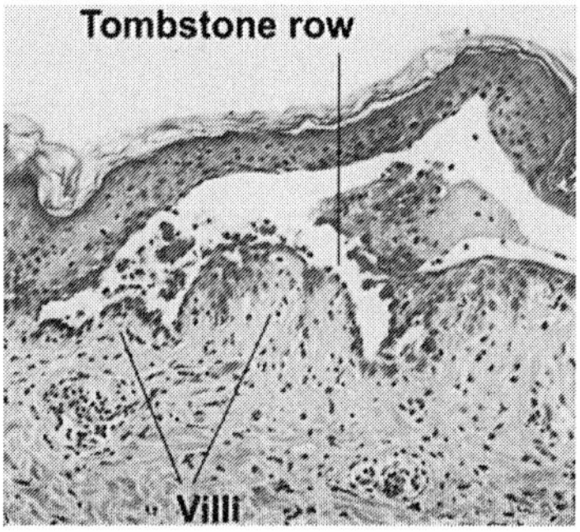

Coming back to the question:

- *Both assertion and reason are true but 'row of tombstones' does not explain suprabasal slitting in pemphigus vulgaris.*

6. A 30 years old male patient had lesions on the trunk, bilaterally. The lesions were minimally pruritic in nature and were having scales at the periphery. Which of the following set of statements is true for the given case?

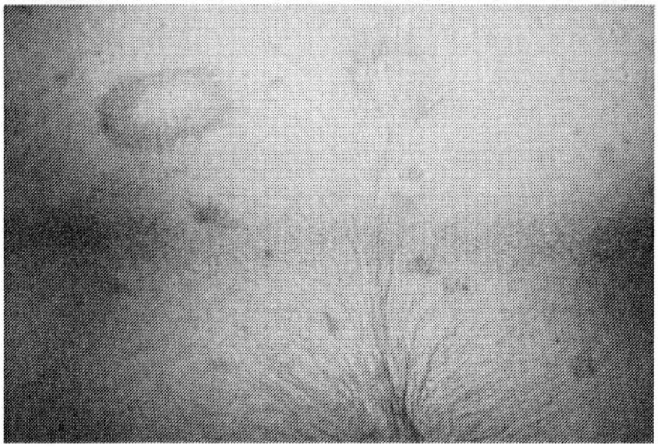

A. Flexor aspect, Collarette of scales, Lichen planus
B. Christmas tree pattern, Wickham's striae, Pityriasis rosea
C. Christmas tree pattern, Collarette of scales, Pityriasis rosea
D. Cigarette paper scales, Wickham's striae, Lichen planus

Key points about Lichen planus:

- *The lesions are faintly erythematous to violaceous flat topped sometimes with central umbilication.*
- *The classic 5Ps of LP are:*
  - *Purple.*
  - *Pruritic.*
  - *Plane.*
  - *Polygonal.*
  - *Papules.*
- *Fine whitish puncta or reticular network known as Wickham striae may be present. These are highly characteristic.*

Key points about Pityriasis rosea:

- *PR is a mild self-limited eruption seen predominantly in adolescents and* ***young*** *adults during the spring and fall.*
- *The disease typically begins with a solitary macule that heralds the eruption (called the herald spot/patch), which is usually a salmon-colored macule.*
- *This initial lesion enlarges over a few days to become a patch with a* ***Collarette*** *of fine scale just inside the well-demarcated border.*
- *About 1-2 weeks after the herald patch is seen, the generalized eruption appears, although it has been known to occur from hours to 3 months later.*
- *It consists of salmon-colored macules or patches, 0.5-1.5 cm in diameter, with a Collarette scale, often described as having a* ***cigarette*** *paper like appearance.*
- *The long axes of the lesions are oriented in a parallel fashion along cleavage lines, giving the classic* ***Christmas*** *tree pattern.*
- *These secondary lesions* ***most*** *commonly occur on the* ***trunk****, the abdomen, the back, and the proximal upper extremities.*
- ***Pruritus*** *occurs in 75% of patients and is severe in 25%.*

Coming back to the question:

- *A 30 years old male with lesions on the trunk (bilaterally), which are minimally pruritic in nature and having scales at the periphery suggest the diagnosis of Pityriasis rosea.*

ANESTHESIA

1. A 55 years old male patient was intubated after acute pancreatitis related complications. His total body weight is 70 kg.

The ventilator settings are as follows:

Tidal Volume of 420 ml,

Respiratory rate of 14/minute,

FiO_2 of 90%,

Positive End Expiratory Pressure/PEEP of 12 cm H_2O.

Arterial blood gas/ABG analysis showed:

sPO_2 of 100%,

pO_2 of 110 mm Hg,

pCO_2 of 48 mm Hg and

pH of 7.33.

What is the best next step in management?

A. Increase tidal volume
B. Increase respiratory rate
C. Increase PEEP to14 cm H_2O
D. Reduce FiO_2

Clinical complication developed in this case is ARDS.

Key points about Mechanical ventilation:

- *The need for mechanical ventilation is one of the* ***most*** *common causes of admission to the intensive care unit.*
- *It is imperative to understand some basic terms to understand mechanical ventilation.*
- *Ventilation:*
    - o *Exchange of gases between the lungs and the air (ambient or delivered by a ventilator), in other words, it is the process of moving air in and out of the lungs.*
    - o *Its most important effect is the removal of carbon dioxide from the body, not on increasing blood oxygen content.*

- *Ventilation is measured as minute ventilation in the clinical setting, and it is calculated as respiratory rate (RR) × Tidal volume (TV).*
- *In a mechanically ventilated patient, the carbon dioxide content of the blood can be modified by the TV or the RR.*

- *Oxygenation:*
  - *Interventions that provide greater oxygen supply to the lungs, thus the circulation.*
  - *In a mechanically ventilated patient, this can be achieved by increasing the fraction of inspired oxygen (FiO_2) or the positive end-expiratory pressure (PEEP).*
- *PEEP:*
  - *The positive pressure that will remain in the airways at the end of the respiratory cycle (end of exhalation) is greater than the atmospheric pressure in mechanically ventilated patients.*
- *Tidal volume: Volume of air moved in or out of lungs in each respiratory cycle.*
- *FiO_2: Percentage of oxygen in the air mixture that is delivered to the patient.*
- *Flow: Speed in liters per minute at which the ventilator delivers breath.*
- *Compliance:*
  - *Change in volume divided by the change in pressure.*
  - *In respiratory physiology, total compliance is a mix of lung and chest wall compliance as these two factors cannot be separated.*
- *Assist Control Ventilation (AC):*
  - *AC is when the ventilator will assist the patient by delivering support for every breath the patient takes (that is the assist part), and the ventilator will have control over the respiratory rate.*
  - *In AC, if the rate is set at 12 and the patient breathes at 18, the ventilator will assist with the 18 breaths, but if the rate drops to 8, the ventilator will take over control of the respiratory rate and deliver 12 breaths in a minute.*
- *Four settings can be easily adjusted in the ventilator (RR, TV, PEEP and FiO_2).*

- *The volume delivered by the ventilator in each breath in assist control will always be the same, regardless of the breath being initiated by the patient or the ventilator, and regardless of compliance, peal, or plateau pressures in the lung.*
- *Initial ventilator management in ARDS:*
  - o *The **most** common ventilator mode to use in a newly intubated patient is AC.*
  - o *The AC mode provides **good** comfort and easy control of some of the most important physiologic parameters.*
  - o *AC mode is used initially with a TV of 6 mL/kg ideal body weight (equals to 420 mL in a 70 kg person as given in the question); RR of 25/minute, flow rate of 60 L/minute, FiO_2 of 100% and a PEEP of 15 cm H_2O.*
  - o *It is started with a FiO_2 of 100% and titrated down guided by pulse oximetry or ABG, depending upon the case.*
  - o *Once oxygen saturation is >90%, FiO_2 is **decreased**.*
  - o *Then, PEEP is decreased in 2.5 cm H_2O increments as tolerated to find the least PEEP associated with an arterial oxygen saturation of 90% on an FiO_2 of ≤60%.*
  - o *The RR is increased up to 35/minute to achieve a pH of >7.15, or until the expiratory flow tracing shows end-expiratory flow.*

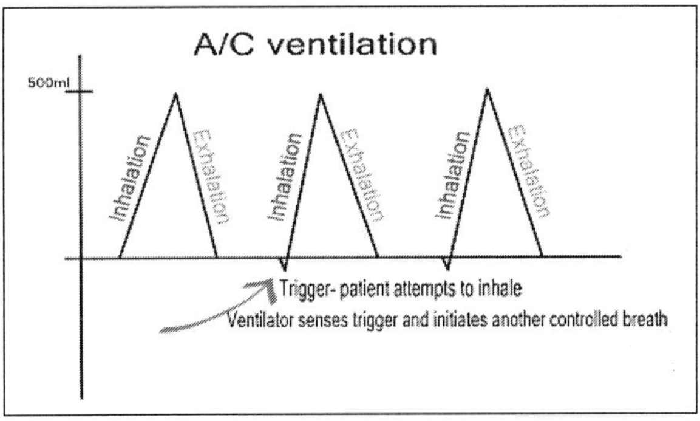

Coming back to the question:

- *We discussed that once oxygen saturation is >90%, FiO_2 is decreased. As saturation is 100% in the given question, so next best step in the management is to reduce the FiO_2; later on we can also reduce the PEEP as well to a level where arterial oxygen saturation* *stays 90% on an FiO_2 of ≤60%. RR need not be increased as the pH given in the question is 7.33 (we discussed that the RR is increased up to 35/minute to achieve a pH of >7.15).*

2. Which of the following statements are true for quality cardiopulmonary resuscitation?

I. Chest compressions at 100-120/minute
II. Ventilation at 22-25/minute
III. Allow full recoil after each compression
IV. In adults, depth of chest compression should be 5-6 cms

Lead – Choose the best answer from the codes given below:

A. I and II
B. I, II and III
C. I, III and IV
D. I, II, III and IV

Let's discuss the options:

Option	*Statement*	*Remarks*
I	Chest compressions at 100-120/minute	• True statement. • After advanced airway (i.e., endotracheal tube, Laryngeal mask airway or combitube), compressions will be continued at the rate of **100** compressions/ minute and breathing at a rate of 8-10 breaths/minute with no synchronization, i.e., no pause for ventilation. • The aim is uninterrupted compressions.
II	Ventilation at 22-25/minute	• False statement. • Ventilation rate should **not** exceed more than **12** breaths/ minute as high rate (more ventilation) will increase intrathoracic pressure which decreases venous return thereby decreasing cardiac output and hence coronary and cerebral perfusion.

Contd.

III	Allow full recoil after each compression	• True statement. • During massage, compression-relaxation (chest recoil) should be **equal**.
IV	In adults, depth of chest compression should be 5-6 cms	• True statement. • CPR is done in supine position. • The rescuer stands (or bend on knee if the victim is on the floor) on side (usually right side), lock one hand over other and provide compression over the lower third of sternum (2 fingers above xiphoid process). • The force generated during massage should be able to depress sternum by 1.5-2 inches/**5** cm (about 1/3rd of chest wall diameter).

Coming back to the question:

- *Ventilation rate in CPR should not exceed 12 breaths/minute.*

RADIOLOGY

1. Banana sign on antenatal USG is seen in:

A. Down syndrome
B. Omphalocele
C. Spina bifida
D. Anencephaly

Let's discuss the options:

Option	*Statement*	*Remarks*
a	Down syndrome	• **Nuchal translucency:** Thickness depends on the size of the fetus (CRL/Crown Rump Length). But in general it is considered **abnormal** if >3 mm. • There is evidence that the inclusion of nasal bone measurement **improves** the specificity of 1st trimester data. • Ductus venosus flow is another parameter that has been reported to **further** increase the sensitivity of 1st trimester screening.
b	Omphalocele	• Omphalocele, also known as exomphalos is a congenital midline abdominal wall defect at the base of the umbilical cord insertion, with herniation of gut out of the fetal abdomen. • Antenatal USG shows multiple bowel **loops** (and on occasion liver) herniate into a membrane-covered defect (i.e., not free-flowing) and are usually seen as hyperechogenic content (non-fluent filled bowel).
c	Spina bifida	• **Lemon sign:** It is considered to have a strong association with spina bifida. • **Banana** sign: The appearance of the cerebellum wrapped around the medulla as part of a Chiari malformation.

Contd.

		• These are the 2 intracranial sonographic findings. • Notably, closed and skin covered spinal lesions typically do **not** have any associated cranial abnormality. • A normal cranial ultrasound therefore does **not** exclude a neural tube defect.
d	Anencephaly	• Anencephaly may be sonographically detectable as **early** as 11 weeks. • Ultrasound can be a non-invasive, cost-effective, and fast method to detect anencephaly and has an accuracy of approximately **100%** at 14 weeks. • **No** parenchymal tissue is seen above the orbits and the calvarium is **absent**; parts of the occipital bone and midbrain may be present. • **Less** than expected value for the CRL. • A '**frog** eye' or 'Mickey **mouse**' appearance may be seen when seen in the coronal plane due to **absent** cranial bone and/or bulging brain and bulging orbits.

Coming back to the question:

- *Banana sign is seen in spinal bifida and/or Chiari II malformation.*

2. Study the given MRCP image and make a diagnosis:

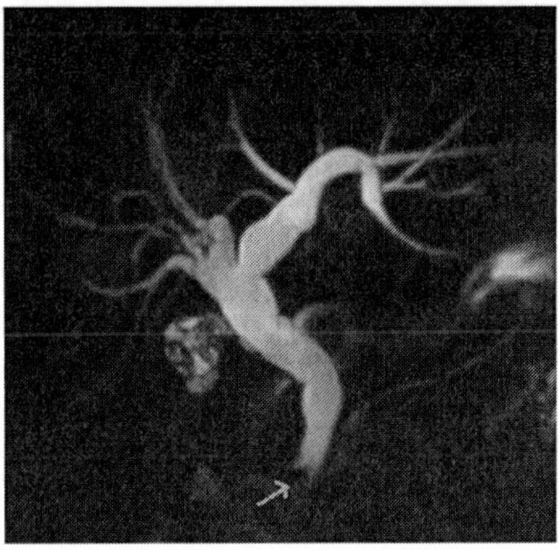

A. Gallbladder stone
B. Common bile duct stricture
C. Common bile duct stone
D. Chronic pancreatitis

Let's discuss the options:

Option	*Statement*	*Remarks*
a	Gallbladder stone	• Ultrasound is considered the **gold** standard for detecting gallstones. • Highly reflective echogenous focus within gallbladder lumen, normally with prominent posterior acoustic shadowing regardless of pathological type (acoustic **shadowing** is independent of the composition and calcium content). • Gravity-dependent movement is often seen with a change of patient position (the rolling **stone** sign).
b	Common bile duct stricture	• As far as assessing the morphology of the stricture (benign/malignant), modalities that image the lumen (ERCP, MRCP, CT intravenous cholangiograms) are **best**, whereas to assess for associated features (pointing to a cause like chronic pancreatitis, previous cholecystetcomy etc.), USG or CT/MRI are **better**.
c	Common bile duct stone	• MRCP (Magnetic Resonance Cholangiopancreatography) has largely ERCP (Endoscopic Retrograde Cholangiopancreatography) as the **gold** standard for diagnosis of choledocholithiasis, able to achieve similar sensitivity (90-94%) and specificity (95-99%) **without** ionizing radiation, intravenous contrast, or the complication rate inherent in ERCP. • Filling **defect** are seen within the biliary tree on thin cross-sectional T2 weighted imaging.

Contd.

d	Chronic pancreatitis	• Late MRI findings include parenchymal atrophy or enlargement, pseudocyst formation and dilatation and beading of the pancreatic duct often with intraductal calcifications, could give a 'chain of **lakes**' appearance.

Coming back to the question:

- *Filling defect in CBD on MRCP, suggest the possibility of CBD stone.*

PSYCHIATRY

1. Which of the following is included in the criterion for dependence syndrome?

I. Tolerance
II. Gradually increased dose of drug intake over time
III. Consumption despite physical harm
IV. Prefers substance over other activities

Lead – Choose the best answer from the codes given below:

A. I and II
B. II and III
C. I, II and III
D. I, II, III and IV

Let's discuss the options:

Option	***Statement***	***Remarks***
I	Tolerance	• True statement. • Dependence should be suspected if there is evidence of **tolerance**, such that increased **doses** of the psychoactive substance are required in order to achieve effects originally produced by lower doses (clear examples of this are found in the alcohol- and opiate-dependent individuals who may take daily doses that are sufficient to incapacitate or kill non-tolerant users).
II	Gradually increased dose of substance intake over time	• True statement.

Contd.

III	Consumption despite physical harm	• True statement. • Persisting with the substance use despite clear evidence of overtly **harmful** consequences, such as harm to the liver through excessive drinking, depressive mood states consequent to periods of heavy substance use, or drug-related impairment of cognitive functioning; efforts should be made to determine that the user was actually, or could be expected to be, aware of the nature and extent of the harm.
IV	Prefers substance over other activities	• True statement. • Progressive **neglect** of alternative pleasures or interests because of psychoactive substance use, increased amount of time necessary to obtain or take the substance or to recover from its effects.

Coming back to the question:

- *Dependence syndrome include tolerance to the psychoactive substance so that patient requires increased dose of substance, consumption despite physical harm and prefers substance over other activities.*

2. SCOFF questionnaire is used for assessing:

A. Mental health
B. Behavioural disorders
C. Sexual disorders
D. Eating disorders

Key points about SCOFF questionnaire:

- *The SCOFF questionnaire is a simple, five-question screening measure to assess the possible presence of an eating disorder*
- *It was developed in the United Kingdom by Morgan and colleagues in 1999.*
- *The SCOFF questionnaire utilizes an acronym (Sick, Control, One, Fat, Food).*

- *Answering 'yes' to two or* ***more*** *of the following questions indicates a possible case of anorexia nervosa, bulimia nervosa, or other eating disorder:*
    - o *Do you make yourself* ***S****ick (induce vomiting) because you feel uncomfortably full?*
    - o *Do you worry you have lost* ***C****ontrol over how much you eat?*
    - o *Have you recently lost more than* ***O****ne stone (approximately fifteen pounds) in a 3 months' period?*
    - o *Do you believe yourself to be* ***F****at when others say you are too thin?*
    - o *Would you say that* ***F****ood dominates your life?*

Coming back to the question:

- *SCOFF questionnaire is used for assessing eating disorders.*

3. A patient had sadness of mood since past few months along with decreased personal hygiene. On examination, his thoughts were like: I am dead, my brain is empty, how will I eat. Such delusions are an example of:

A. Persecutory delusion
B. Bizarre delusion
C. Nihilistic delusion
D. Cotard delusion

Let's discuss the options:

Option	*Statement*	*Remarks*
a	Persecutory delusion	• A persecutory delusion or persecution complex is a delusional condition in which the affected person believes that harm is going to occur to oneself by a persecutor, despite a clear lack of evidence. • The person may believe that they are being targeted by an individual or a group of people. • The delusion can be found in multitude of disorders, being more usual in psychotic disorders, such as schizophrenia, schizoaffective disorder and delusional disorder.

Contd.

b	Bizarre delusion	• A bizarre delusion, by contrast, is something that could **never** happen in real life, such as being cloned by aliens or having thoughts broadcast on TV.
c	Nihilistic delusion	• These are seen in depression (**sadness** of mood). • Nihilistic delusions are the delusion that things (or everything, including the self) do not exist; a sense that everything is unreal. • Nihilistic delusions are characterized by the delusional belief of being **dead**, decomposed or annihilated, having lost one's own internal **organs** or even not existing as a human being. • The patient believes he no longer exits, that his mind or a part of the body is missing, or the world itself has ceased to be. • This delusion takes a variety of forms. • My brain has rotted away. • I died twenty-five years ago and now only my spirit remains. • I lost my left eye in a car accident. • My whole family is dead and gone and I haven't a friend left alive. • This is a dream world, all shadow and no substance. • I am only an empty shell. • I have no stomach, no liver, no genital organs.
d	Cotard delusion	• Cotard's syndrome is a relatively rare condition that was first described by Dr. Jules Cotard in 1882.

Contd.

		• Cotard's syndrome/Walking corpse syndrome comprises any one of a series of delusions that range from a belief that one has **lost** organs, blood, or body parts to insisting that one has lost one's soul or is **dead**.

Coming back to the question:

- *Clinical presentation is indicative of depression and delusion discussed in question is nihilistic delusion.*

4. All of the following are causes of reversible dementia EXCEPT:

A. Multi-infarct dementia
B. Lewy body disease
C. Hypothyroidism
D. Normal pressure hydrocephalus

Let's discuss the options:

Option	*Statement*	*Remarks*
a	Multi-infarct dementia/ MID	• Multi-infarct dementia is the **second** most common cause of dementia seen in 10-15% of all cases, though some studies indicate that MID is probably far more common in India. • It is also one of the **most** important **treatable** causes of dementia. • Occurrence of multiple cerebral infarction can lead to a progressive disruption of brain function, leading to dementia. • There is an abrupt onset, acute exacerbations and stepwise clinical deterioration (step-ladder pattern). • The course is fluctuating, with history of previous stroke or transient ischemic attacks/TIA. • There is presence of hypertension (**most** commonly) or any other significant cardiovascular disease.

Contd.

b	Lewy body disease	• Lewy body dementia is now believed to be the second **most** common cause of the degenerative dementias, accounting for about 4% of all the dementias. • There is fluctuating cognitive impairment over weeks or months, with involvement of memory and higher cortical functions (such as language, visuospatial ability, praxis and reasoning). • Lucid intervals can be present in between fluctuations. • Recurrent and detailed visual hallucinations are present. • Spontaneous extrapyramidal or parkinsonian symptoms such as rigidity and tremors.
c	Hypothyroidism	• Hypothyroid dementia has been considered one of the **most** important **treatable** causes of dementia, second only to toxic dementias. • Although it accounts for less than 1% of dementias, hypothyroidism should be suspected in every patient of dementia.
d	Normal pressure hydrocephalus	• Some underlying causes of dementia are treatable (reversible dementias), for example, treatment of hypertension in MID, thyroxin replacement in hypothyroid dementia, shunting in **hydrocephalic** dementia, levodopa in parkinsonism, and removal of the toxic agent in toxic dementias.

Coming back to the question:

- *Lewy body disease is an example of irreversible dementia.*

5. La belle indifference is seen in:

A. Mania

B. Depression

C. Schizophrenia

D. Conversion disorder

Key points about La belle indifference:

- *One of the feature of dissociative (conversion) disorders is la belle indifference, which is a lack of concern towards the symptoms, despite the apparent severity of the disability produced.*
- *Although earlier thought to be* ***hallmark*** *of dissociative (conversion) disorders, it is now known to be present even in physical illnesses.*
- *In addition, it is* ***not*** *always present in dissociative (conversion) disorders.*

Coming back to the question:

- *La belle indifference is a feature of dissociative (conversion) disorders.*

ORTHOPEDICS

1. A patient had an injury to some part of humerus. On clinical examination, patient was unable to flex the distal interphalangeal joint of 4th and 5th fingers and was not able to hold a card between fingers. Which part of humerus is injured?

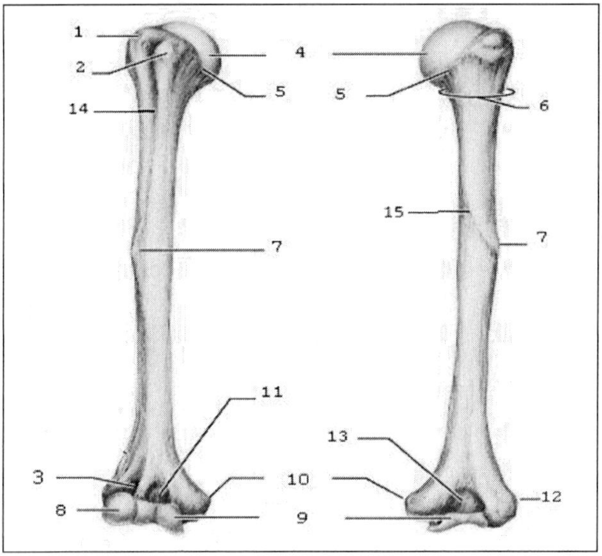

A. 12 B. 10
C. 15 D. 6

Let's discuss the options:

Option	*Statement*	*Remarks*
a	12	• The landmark is lateral epicondyle. • **No** nerve is usually (directly) injured in fracture of lateral epicondyle though tardy ulnar nerve palsy can be seen in non-union fracture lateral epicondyle with cubital valgus deformity.

Contd.

b	10	• The landmark is medial epicondyle and the nerve, which can injure is ulnar nerve. • The ulnar nerve is most often injured as it lies behind the medial epicondyle of the humerus. • Muscles supplied by the ulnar nerve may be paralyzed depending upon the level of injury. • **High** ulnar nerve palsy: The injury is proximal to the elbow and causes paralysis of all the muscles supplied by the ulnar nerve in the forearm (FCU, **medial** half of FDP) and hand (hypothenar muscles, adductor pollicis, all interossei and medial two lumbricals). • **FDP:** It is the flexor of distal inter-phalangeal/DIP joints. • **Low** ulnar nerve palsy: The injury is in the distal third of the forearm and there is sparing of forearm muscles but the muscles of the hand are paralyzed. • **Card** test is positive. The patient is asked to grip a sheet of paper forcefully between the thumbs and index fingers while the examiner tries to pull it away. • In ulnar nerve palsy, it can be pulled away easily suggesting weakness of palmar interossei. • Egawa test and book test is also **positive**.
c	15	• The landmark is radial groove and the nerve, which can injure is radial nerve. • **High** radial nerve palsy: This occurs if the nerve is injured in the radial groove. • In this type, all the muscles supplied by the radial nerve **except** the triceps and anconeus are paralyzed.

Contd.

		• Occasionally, the radial nerve may be injured still higher up, in which case even the triceps may be paralyzed. • This is called **very** high radial nerve palsy. • **Lower** radial nerve palsy: This occurs if the nerve is injured around the elbow so that the muscles supplied by the radial nerve in the distal arm (brachioradialis, ECRL and ECRB are spared).
d	6	• The landmark is surgical neck humerus and the nerve, which can injure is axillary nerve. • The axillary nerve arises from the posterior cord of the brachial plexus and curves backwards on the lower border of the subscapularis. • It crosses the quadrangular space and comes to lie on the medial side of the surgical neck of the humerus, medial and inferior to the capsule of the shoulder joint. • Here it divided into anterior and posterior branches. • The posterior branch supplies the teres minor and posterior part of the deltoid and terminates as the cutaneous nerve which supplies the skin over the lower-half of the deltoid. • The anterior branch continues horizontally between the deltoid and the surgical neck of the humerus, and supplies the rest of the deltoid. • Axillary nerve palsy manifest as paralysis of deltoid and Regiment badge sign.

Coming back to the question:

- *Ulnar nerve is injured in fracture of medial epicondyle. Patient cannot flex the DIP of 4th and 5th finger. Card test is also positive.*

2. A young male with Road Traffic Accident presented to the Emergency room. On examination he was found to have fracture of femur. At presentation his vitals were stable but after 12 hours he developed tachypnea, disorientation and rash in chest and axilla. Most likely diagnosis:

A. Deep venous thrombosis
B. Pulmonary embolism
C. Fat embolism
D. Adult respiratory distress syndrome

Let's discuss the options:

Option	*Statement*	*Remarks*
a, b	Deep venous thrombosis, Pulmonary embolism	• DVT is a **common** complication associated with lower limb injuries and with spinal injuries. • Immobilization following trauma leads to venous stasis which results in thrombosis of veins. • DVT can be recognised as early as 48 hours after the injury. • Leg swelling and calf tenderness are usual signs of DVT. • DVT proximal to the knee is a **common** cause of life threatening complication of pulmonary embolism/PE. • Embolism occurs, usually 4-5 days after the injury. • PE is suspected if the patient develops tachypnea and dyspnoea, usually 4-5 days after the accident. • There may be chest pain or hemoptysis.

Contd.

c	Fat embolism	• Fat embolism is **more** common following severe injuries with multiple fractures and fractures of **major** bones. • Symptoms are evident in a **day** or so after the injury. • Presenting features are in the form of two, more or less distinct types: (i) cerebral; and (ii) pulmonary. • In the cerebral type, the patient becomes drowsy, restless and **disoriented** and gradually goes into a state of coma. • In the pulmonary type, **tachypnea** and tachycardia are the more prominent features. • The other common feature of fat embolism is a petechial **rash**, usually on the front of the neck, anterior axillary folds, chest or conjunctiva.
d	Adult respiratory distress syndrome	• ARDS can be sequelae of trauma with subsequent shock. • The onset is usually 24 hours after the injury. • The patient develops tachypnea and laboured breathing. • X-ray chest shows **diffuse** pulmonary infiltrates.

Coming back to the question:

- *If a patient develops tachypnea, disorientation and rash (in chest and axilla) after 12 hours of fracture of femur, the possibility of fat embolism should be kept in mind.*

3. A young boy of 16 years of age presented to the Orthopedics OPD with a growth arising from lower end of right femur. Growth was present since last 3 years. X-ray was done as shown below. Which of the following statement is true regarding malignant transformation of the growth?

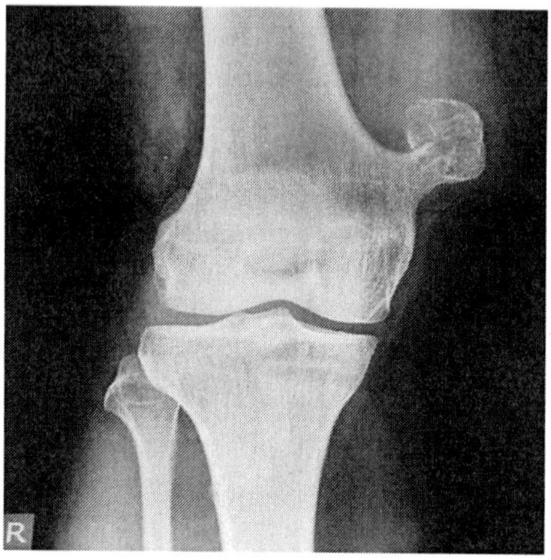

A. Such a growth never turns malignant
B. If the marrow of the growth connects with the marrow of the primary bone
C. MRI showing hyaline cap of >2 cm after skeletal maturity
D. If the swelling starts moving towards the joint

Key points about Osteochondroma/Exostosis:

- *This is the **most common** benign 'tumour' of the bone.*
- *It is **not** a true neoplasm since its growth stops with cessation of growth at the epiphyseal plate.*
- *It is a result of an aberration at the growth plate, where a few cells from the plate grow centrifugally as a separate lump of bone.*
- *Though the tumour originates at the growth plate, it gets 'left behind' as the bone grows in length, and thus comes to lie at the metaphysis.*
- *The stalk and part of the head of the tumour are made up of mature bone, but the tip is covered with cartilage.*
- *Malignant transformation occurs in the cartilage cap (chondrosarcoma).*
- *A rapid increase in the size of the tumour and appearance of pain in a hitherto painless swelling may be **suggestive** of malignant transformation.*
- *MRI is the **best** imaging modality to assess cartilage thickness (and thus assessing for malignant transformation).*

- *A cartilage cap of over **1.5** cm in thickness after skeletal maturity is suspicious for malignant degeneration, while the cartilage cap may be seen up to 3 cm in thickness in young patients.*

Coming back to the question:

- *A cartilage cap of over **1.5** cm in thickness (after skeletal maturity) is suspicious for malignant degeneration in an exostosis.*

4. A patient had a fall on ground over his shoulder, following which he developed pain and swelling over shoulder joint. X-ray of the patient is shown below. Which ligaments are torn in the given case?

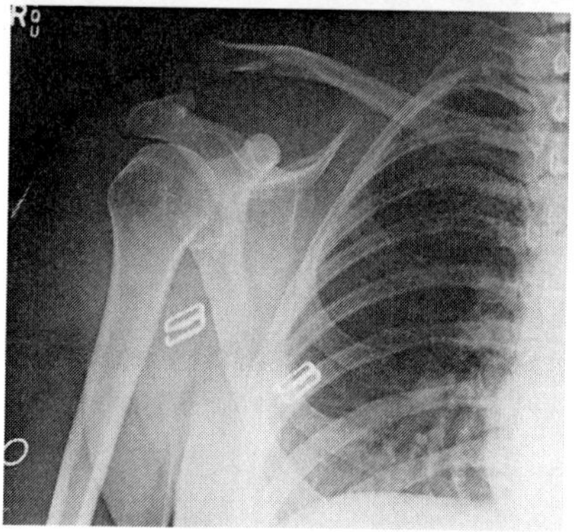

A. Acromioclavicular ligament

B. Coracoclavicular ligament

C. Both acromioclavicular and coracoclavicular ligaments

D. Corcohumeral ligament

Key points about Acromioclavicular joint injury:

- *Subluxation or dislocation of the acromioclavicular joint is an uncommon injury, caused by a fall on the outer prominence of the shoulder.*
- *The injury may result in a partial or complete rupture of the acromio-clavicular (AC) or coracoclavicular (CC) ligaments.*
- *Pain and swelling localized to the acromioclavicular joint indicates an injury to this joint.*
- *Grades:*
    - o *Grade I: Minimal strain to the AC ligament and joint capsule.*

- o *Grade II: Rupture of AC ligament and joint capsule.*
- o *Grade III:*
  - ♦ *Rupture of AC ligament, joint capsule and CC ligament.*
  - ♦ *The lateral end of the clavicle may be unusually prominent.*

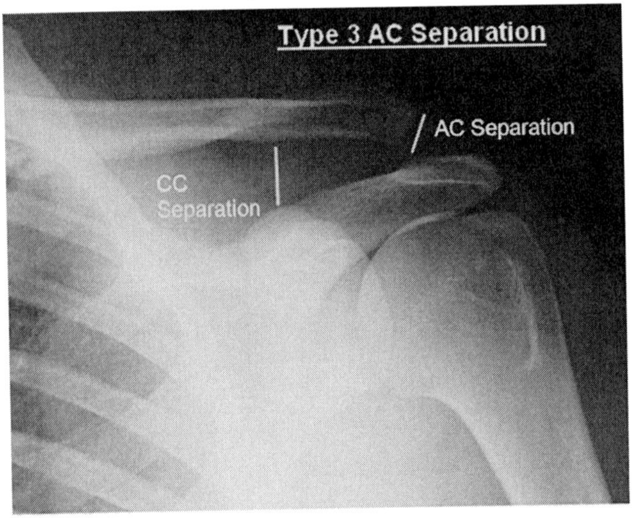

Coming back to the question:

- *In grade III acromioclavicular joint injury, both AC ligament and CC ligaments are torn.*

5. A patient with Road Traffic Accident presented to the Emergency department with fracture of pelvis. He was hypotensive. What should be done first?

A. Immediate external fixation

B. Blood transfusion

C. Tie a bedsheet around pelvis

D. Prepare for internal fixation

Key points about Management of Unstable pelvic fractures:

- *With any severely injured patient, the first step is to make sure that the airway is clear and ventilation is unimpaired.*
- *Resuscitation must be started immediately and active bleeding controlled.*

- *For patients with very severe injuries, **early external** fixation is one of the **most** effective ways of reducing hemorrhage and counteracting shock.*
- *Application of external fixator for major pelvic trauma is an important component of many resuscitation protocols, with the goal of stabilizing the pelvis to control hemorrhage, decrease blood transfusion rates and improve survival rates.*
- *External fixation:*
  - o *This is a reliable and comfortable method.*
  - o *Two or three pins threaded at the tip (Schanz pin) are inserted in the anterior part of the wing of the iliac bone on each side.*

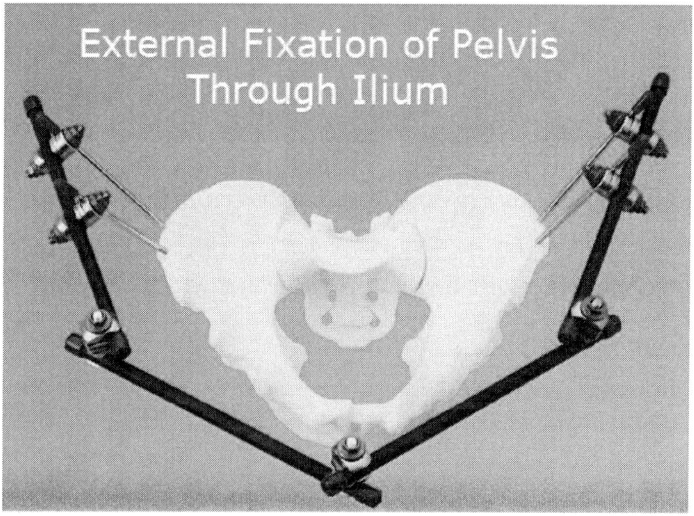

  - o *After reduction of the displacement by manual pressure, the pins are clamped to a metal rod or frame placed transversely over the front of the pelvis.*

Coming back to the question:

- *Immediate external fixation stabilizes the fracture and controls further bleeding in unstable pelvic fractures.*

6. A patient sustained injury to chest and had ribs fractures. Chest X-ray was done. Identify the ribs fractured:

A. 5th, 6th B. 6th, 7th
C. 7th, 8th D. 8th, 9th

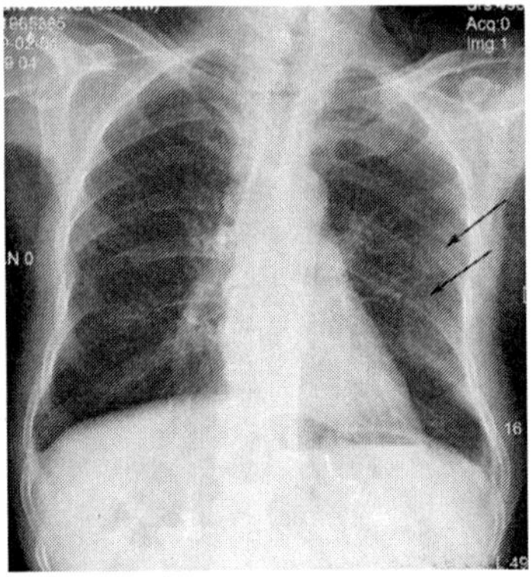

Key points about counting ribs on Chest X-ray:

- *Identify the transverse process of the first thoracic vertebra and the articulating rib, which is the first rib. First rib can be identified easily. It is broad as compared to other ribs.*
- *Count downward.*
- *Anterior ends are curved and lateral (numbering in blue).*
- *Posterior ends are straight and near spine (numbering in yellow).*
- *Anterior end of 7th rib touches the midclavicular line.*

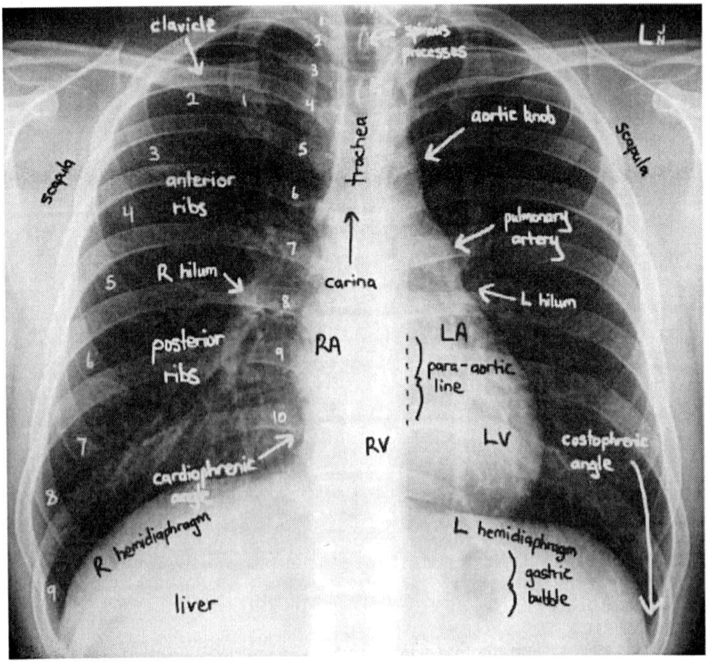

Coming back to the question:

- *X-ray given the questions shows fracture of 6th and 7th ribs.*

7. An 8 years old girl presented with painful swelling over upper limbs and lower limbs. X-ray of the pelvis with both the hips was done. She is also having hypothyroidism. Skin rash was seen. Bone scan showed increased uptake in humerus, femurs, skull, ribs etc. Most likely diagnosis:

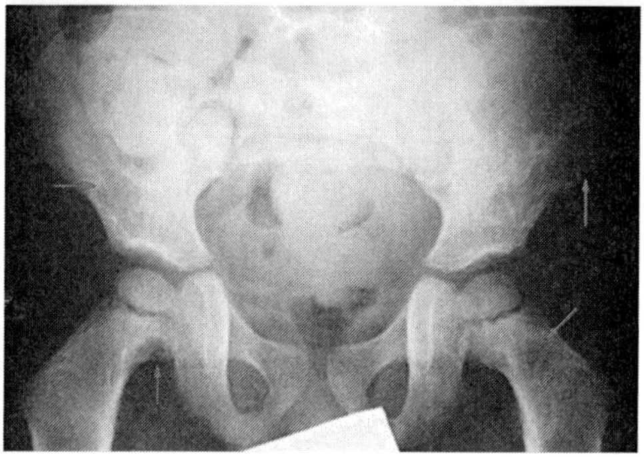

A. Langerhans cell histiocytosis
B. Papillary carcinoma thyroid with bony metastasis
C. McCune Albright syndrome
D. Neurofibroma with bony involvement

Let's discuss the options:

Option	*Statement*	*Remarks*
a	Langerhans cell histiocytosis	• LCH provokes a non-specific inflammatory response, which includes fever, lethargy and weight loss. • Organ involvement can also cause more specific symptoms. • **Bone:** The **most** frequently seen symptom in both unifocal and multifocal disease is **painful** bone **swelling**. • The skull is most frequently affected, followed by the long bones of the upper **extremity** and flat bones.

Contd.

		• Infiltration in hands and feet is unusual. • **Osteolytic** lesions can lead to pathological fractures. • **Skin:** Commonly seen are a **rash** which varies from scaly erythematous lesions to red papules pronounced in intertriginous areas. • Up to 80% of LCH patients have extensive eruptions on the scalp. • **Lymph node:** Enlargement of the liver in 20%, spleen in 30% and lymph nodes in 50% of Histiocytosis cases. • **Endocrine glands:** Hypothalamic pituitary axis commonly involved. • Diabetes insipidus is **most** common. • **Anterior** pituitary hormone deficiency is usually permanent. • **Bone scan:** There is a variable appearance on bone scintigraphy with lesions showing an **increased** or decreased tracer uptake depending upon the histological picture.
b	Papillary thyroid carcinoma/ PTC with bony metastasis	• PTC presents as soft/hard/firm, solid/ cystic, solitary/multinodular thyroid swelling. • Bony metastases are much **less** common in PTC (1-7%). • Often discrete lymph nodes in the neck (40%) are palpable.
c	McCune Albright syndrome/MAS	• The Orthopedic entity associated with MAS is polyostotic fibrous dysplasia/ FD. • X-ray of FD show radiolucent 'cystic' areas in the metaphysis or shaft;

Contd.

		because they contain fibrous tissue with diffuse spots of immature bone, the lucent patches typically have a slightly hazy or 'ground-glass' appearance. • The weight-bearing bones may be bent, and one of the **classic** features is the 'shepherd's crook' deformity of the proximal femur. • Radioscintigraphy shows **marked** activity of the lesion. • Occasionally the bone disorder is associated with café-au-lait patches on the skin and (in girls) precocious sexual development.
d	Neurofibroma with bony involvement	• It is a benign tumour arising from connective tissue of the nerve containing ectodermal neural and mesodermal connective tissue component. • Patient present with mild pain/painless swelling usually in subcutaneous or cutaneous plane with tingling, numbness or paresthesia along the distribution of the nerve.

Coming back to the question:

- *Painful swelling over upper limbs and lower limbs, hypothyroidism, skin rash, osteolytic lesions on X-rays and increased uptake on bone scan suggest the possibility of Langerhans cell histiocytosis.*

PEDIATRICS

1. An 18 months old child had history of loose motions and vomiting for 3 days. He presented to the emergency in a state of poor sensorium. Which of the following complications can be seen in this case?

I. Severe dehydration
II. Cerebral venous thrombosis
III. Hemolytic uremic syndrome
IV. Hyponatremia

Lead – Choose the best answer from the codes given below:

A. I and II
B. II and III
C. I, II and III
D. I, II, III and IV

Let's discuss the options:

Option	*Statement*	*Remarks*
I	Severe dehydration	• True statement. • In severe dehydration, the child passes '**too many**' loose motions and has severe vomiting to the extent that nothing is retained and the oral intake becomes virtually impracticable. • Child becomes lethargic/unconscious. • Eyes are very sunken and dry. • Tears are **absent.** • On pinching, skin goes back **very** slowly (>2 seconds).
II	Cerebral venous thrombosis	• True statement. • Manifestations secondary to CNS disturbances are prominent in all types of severe dehydration (isotonic, hypotonic and hypertonic).

Contd.

		• Hypertonic dehydration has more of these. • Early irritability, alternating with apathy, may progress to delirium or stupor, lethargy and coma. • Convulsions may occur at any stage. • The high viscosity of blood may cause as serious complication as **cerebral** thrombosis.
III	Hemolytic uremic syndrome	• True statement. • The hemolytic uremic syndrome/**HUS** is an acute disorder characterized by renal failure with or without oligoanuria, microangiopathic hemolytic anemia and thrombocytopenia. • It is the **most** common cause of acute renal failure in young children. • Two broad subgroups have been described. • One form is **not** associated with antecedent diarrhea and is called D-HUS, is **rare** in children. • The other one is **commonly** seen in infants and is associated with a diarrhoeal prodrome. • This is called D+ HUS. • An acute enteritis with diarrhea caused by verocytotoxin producing E. coli 0157:H7 precedes 80% or more of cases of HUS in developed countries. • In the developing countries, the common organism is Shigella dysenteriae type 1 that produces shiga toxin 1.

Contd.

IV	Hyponatremia	• True statement. • Loss of water from child's body causes shrinkage in the volume of the ECF compartment. • In around one-half cases with extensive sodium loss in stools, **hyponatremia** develops as a result of fall in serum and ECF sodium levels. • Since sodium is the major determinant of osmolality, this results in fall osmolality of ECF. • Then follows movement of water from ECF to ICF compartment. • Further shrinkage of the already shrunk ECF compartment volume becomes inevitable. • This is manifested in the form of loss or impairment of skin elasticity.

Coming back to the question:

- *Complications seen in a case of acute severe gastroenteritis are severe dehydration, cerebral thrombosis, HUS and hyponatremia.*

2. Which of the following are included in Nada's minor criterias for diagnosing congenital heart disease?

I. Abnormal second heart sound
II. Diastolic murmur
III. Abnormal chest X-ray
IV. Systolic murmur grade-III

Lead – Choose the best answer from the codes given below:

A. I and III
B. II and III
C. I, II and III
D. I, III and IV

Key points about Nada's criteria:

- *Alexander Nada has given a score for the detection of CHD (congenital heart diseases) on the basis of clinical evaluation very early in 1950s-1960s.*

- *Nada's criteria have four major and five minor components.*
- *Major criteria:*
  - o *Systolic murmur of grade III or more.*
  - o *Diastolic murmurs.*
  - o *Cyanosis.*
  - o *Congestive cardiac failure.*
- *Minor criteria:*
  - o *Systolic murmur of grade <3.*
  - o *Abnormal* ***second*** *heart sound.*
  - o *Abnormal ECG.*
  - o *Abnormal chest* ***X-ray****.*
  - o *Abnormal BP.*
- *There has to be one major* ***or*** *two minor criteria to label CHD.*

Coming back to the question:

- *Among the options given in the questions, abnormal second heart sound and abnormal chest X-ray are considered in Nada's minor criteria.*

3. A 4 years old child presented with high grade fever for 6 days. On examination, conjunctival injection and strawberry tongue was seen. There was peeling of periungual skin. 2D-ECHO revealed coronary artery aneurysm. Most appropriate line of management:

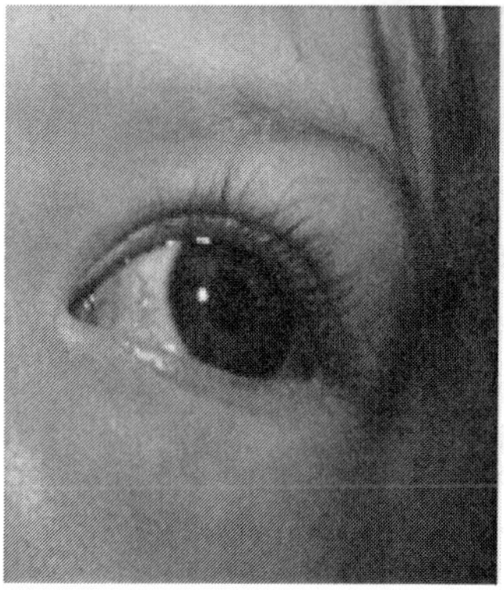

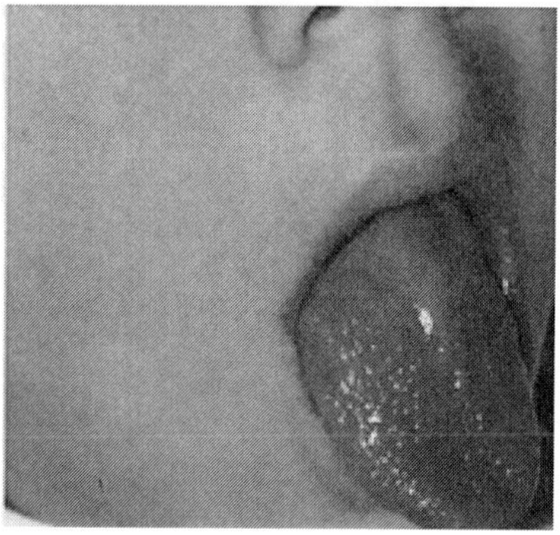

A. Aspirin
B. I/V Immunoglobulin
C. Low molecular weight heparin
D. Dipyridamole

Clinical presentation is indicative of Kawasaki disease.

Key points about Kawasaki disease:

- *Also known as Mucocutaneous lymph node syndrome/Infantile polyarteritis.*
- *First described in 1967 by Prof T Kawasaki of Tokyo, it has emerged as an important cause of vasculitis and heart disease in children.*
- *The disease is characterized by prolonged high pyrexia, conjunctivitis, stomatitis, cervical lymphadenopathy and macular erythema with pronounced reddening of palms and soles and subsequent desquamation of the digits (usually beginning periungually).*
- *Essential diagnostic criteria:*
    - o ***Fever** lasting for a **minimal** of 5 days.*
    - o *Illness not explained by any other known disease process.*
- *Non-essential diagnostic criteria (4 of the 5 features suffice):*
    - o *Bilateral non-purulent conjunctival **injection**.*
    - o *Changes of the mucosa of the oropharynx, including infected pharynx, infected and/or dry fissured lips, **strawberry** tongue.*
    - o *Changes in the peripheral extremities, e.g., edema and/or erythema of hands or feet, desquamation usually beginning **periungually**.*
    - o *Rash (primarily truncal) – polymorphous but non-vesicular.*
    - o *Cervical lymphadenopathy (at **least** one node >1.5 cm).*
- *Cardiac studies must include 2-dimensional echocardiography at time of first presentation and then after 2 weeks for detecting coronary dilatation or **aneurysm**.*
- *Currently the treatment of **choice** is high dose intravenous immunoglobulin. The response is **dramatic**. Moreover, it also prevents coronary vascular involvement.*
- *During the febrile phase, the subject should also be given salicylates/ Aspirin.*

- *If coronary lesions are already present, this therapy with or without dipyridamole needs to be carried on until the coronary involvement has regressed.*
- *Heparin or warfarin therapy may be added in case of large aneurysms.*

Coming back to the question:

- *I/V immunoglobulin is the treatment of choice for Kawasaki disease.*

4. You attended a delivery of a baby with meconium stained amniotic fluid/MSAF. Which of the following statements are true regarding neonatal resuscitation program/NRP?

I. Gentle mouth and nose wiping in vigorous infant with MSAF

II. Positive pressure ventilation in non-vigorous infant with MSAF after initial steps

III. Tracheal suction in non-vigorous infant with MSAF

IV. Intrapartum suctioning should be done before delivery of shoulders

Lead – Choose the best answer from the codes given below:

A. I and II
B. II and III
C. I, II and III
D. I, II, III and IV

Key points about Vigorous infant:

- *Good muscle tone.*
- *Active breathing efforts.*
- *Heart rate > 100 beats/minute.*

Let's discuss the options:

Option	*Statement*	*Remarks*
I	Gentle mouth and nose wiping in vigorous infant with MSAF	• True statement. • Most vigorous newborns do **not** require suctioning at birth. • If necessary, remove secretions by **wiping** the baby's mouth and nose with a cloth.

Contd.

		• Use a bulb syringe when secretions are obstructing the baby's breathing, and for those having difficulty clearing their secretions.
II	Positive pressure ventilation/PPV in non-vigorous infant with MSAF after initial steps	• True statement. • The recent NRP **recommends** against suctioning but favours resuscitation with **PPV** on non-vigorous neonates with MSAF. • This recommendation is aimed to **prevent** delay in resuscitation and **minimize** hypoxia-ischemia often associated with MSAF.
III	Tracheal suction in non-vigorous infant with MSAF	• False statement. • The 2015 NRP recommended that even non-vigorous infants delivered through MSAF did **not** routinely require intubation and tracheal suction. • The aforementioned recommendation of change in practice placed a greater value on **avoiding** the harm of intubation and delaying the establishment of breathing over the undetermined benefits of routine tracheal intubation and suction.
IV	Intrapartum suctioning should be done before delivery of shoulders	• False statement. • Sucking out the baby's mouth and pharynx on the perineum before the delivery of the shoulders makes **no** difference to the outcome of babies with MSAF and is **no** longer recommended.

Coming back to the question:

- *As per NRP guidelines, gentle mouth and nose wiping should be done in vigorous infant with MSAF whereas in non-vigorous infant should be resuscitated with PPV. Tracheal suctioning or intrapartum suctioning is no longer recommended.*